Improving Hospital Care for Persons with Dementia

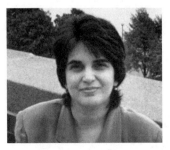

Nina M. Silverstein, Ph.D., is an Associate Professor of Gerontology at the University of Massachusetts Boston, College of Public and Community Service. Since 1984, she has worked closely with the Alzheimer's Association on projects related to patient care, caregiver, and community support. She served as Chairperson of the Massachusetts Statewide Chapter of the Alzheimer's Association and also was a long-time board member for the Council on Aging in Needham, Massachusetts—the first accredited and reaccredited Senior Center in Massachusetts. She is a Fellow of the Gerontological Society of America and active member of the American Society on Aging and the Association for Gerontology in Higher Education.

A graduate of the Heller School, Brandeis University, Nina has been publishing and presenting on aging issues at national conferences since the onset of her career over 20 years ago. She co-authored *Dementia and Wandering Behavior: Concern for the Lost Elder* (Springer Publishing Company), a 2002 recipient of the American Journal of Nursing Book of the Year Award. Nina resides in Needham, Massachusetts with her husband Irwin and has two daughters, Ilana and Julie.

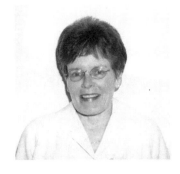

Katie Maslow, M.S.W., is Associate Director for Quality Care Advocacy at the Alzheimer's Association. She directs the Association's ongoing initiative on improving hospital care for people with dementia. Prior to joining the Alzheimer's Association in 1995, Katie was a policy analyst and senior associate at the U.S. Office of Technology Assessment (OTA), a congressional research agency, where she worked on studies of policy issues in aging, Alzheimer's disease, long-term care, and case management. Before coming to OTA in 1983, she worked in nursing home, mental health, and public welfare settings.

Katie has an undergraduate degree from Stanford University and a masters degree in social work from Howard University. She is on the national board of the American Society on Aging and is a member of the American Geriatrics Society, the American Public Health Association, the Gerontological Society of America, and the National Association of Social Workers. She lives in Bethesda, Maryland, with her husband, Harvey Eisen, and has two daughters, Carrie and Gayle.

Improving Hospital Care for Persons with Dementia

Nina M. Silverstein, PhD
Katie Maslow, MSW, Editors
With Foreword by Eric Tangalos, MD

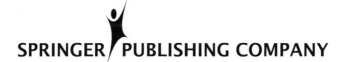

SPRINGER PUBLISHING COMPANY

Springer Publishing Company, Inc.
11 West 42nd Street, 15th Floor
New York, NY 10036-8002

Acquisitions Editor: Helvi Gold
Production Editor: Print Matters
Cover design by Springer Publishing
Compositor: Compset, Inc.

06 07 08 09 10/5 4 3 2 1

Library of Congress Catalogue-in-Publication Data

Improving hospital care for persons with dementia /
Nina M.
Silverstein, Katie Maslow, co-editors.
        p. cm.
   Includes bibliographical references and index.
   ISBN 0-8261-3915-9
   1. Dementia—Patients—Hospital care—United States.
   I. Silverstein,
Nina M.   II. Maslow, Katie.

RC521.I49 2006
362.196'83—dc22

2005054408

ISBN 0-8261-3915-9

Printed in the United States of America by Kase Printing, Inc.

Dedication

This book is dedicated to promoting dignity and safety for people with Alzheimer's disease and other dementing illnesses who may find themselves hospitalized and unable to communicate their pain, suffering, or frustration.

Contents

Contributors

Luis Felipe Amador, MD, is the medical director of the ACE Unit at the University of Texas Medical Branch, Galveston, Texas. He is board certified in internal medicine and geriatric medicine. His professional interests include hospital care of the older adult and geriatric education, especially the education of medical students.

Jackie Beckwith, RN, MSN, is a nurse at Providence St. Vincent Hospice in Oregon. She received her B.S.N. from Oregon Health Sciences University and her MSN from the University of Portland. While working for Providence Milwaukie Hospital, she led efforts to develop a Geriatric Resource Team to improve care for hospitalized elders.

Emily Spilseth Binstadt, MD, is a 2003 graduate of the Brigham and Women's Hospital/Massachusetts General Hospital Harvard Affiliated Emergency Medicine Residency. She is interested in ethics in emergency medicine and is currently pursuing a master's degree at the Harvard School of Public Health and a fellowship in medical education and simulation.

Marie Boltz, MSN, RN, is the director of Practice Initiatives for the John A. Hartford Institute for Geriatric Nursing at New York University. A gerontologic nurse practitioner and licensed nursing home administrator, she has extensive administrative and clinical expertise in the field of dementia care and in multiple practice settings. Her research interests include the maintenance of function in persons with dementia and end-of-life care.

Mary W. Carter, PhD, is an assistant professor of gerontology at West Virginia University School of Medicine's Center on Aging. Prior to joining the Center on Aging, Dr. Carter was a National Institute of Aging Postdoctoral Fellow at the University of Minnesota, Division of Health Services Research. Her research interests include variations in hospital use rates among nursing home residents, organizational and structural determinants of differential quality of care and health outcomes among residents of nursing home facilities, and end-of-life care for residents with Alzheimer's disease.

Frances Conedera, RN, MS, PMHNP, is a psychiatric mental health nurse practitioner in private practice and part-time adjunct faculty at Linfield-Good Samaritan School of Nursing in Oregon. She was project author and co-director for the Alzheimer's Association-funded grant, "Improving Care of Hospitalized Elders with Dementia." Frances received her B.S.N. from Oregon Health Sciences University in 1974, her M.S. from the University of California at San Francisco in 1979, and completed her post-masters nurse practitioner work at Washington State University in 2003.

Charles E. Drebing, PhD, is an assistant professor of psychiatry at the Boston University School of Medicine and the associate director of mental health at the Bedford VA Medical Center. His research interests include family caregiving and healthcare utilization among adults with Alzheimer's disease. He is the coordinator of caregiving research for the Boston University Alzheimer's Disease Core Center and is the principal investigator of the Vulnerable and Isolated Persons (VIP) with Alzheimer's Disease study, funded by the Alzheimer's Association.

Germaine Edinger, MS, has been a Psychiatric Clinical Nurse Specialist for 15 years. She has been involved with North Memorial Health Care's TWICE *(Together We're Improving Care for Elders)* Committee since the onset of the project. In her patient/family consultation practice, she sees many diagnoses of dementia and delirium.

Khama Ennis, MD, MPH, is a second-year emergency medicine resident in the Brigham and Women's Hospital/Massachusetts General Hospital Harvard Affiliated Emergency Medicine Residency. Her specific areas of interest include ethics and geriatrics.

Susan Farrell, MD, is an assistant professor of medicine at Harvard Medical School and attending physician in the Department of Emergency Medicine at Brigham and Women's Hospital. She was a recipient of the Harvard/Hartford Center for Excellence in Geriatrics Junior Faculty Award in 2000–2001, during which time she studied the use of advance directives in elderly emergency department patients.

Patricia Finch Guthrie, PhD, APRN, BC (CNS) is the Director of Clinical Practice, Innovation and Resarch at North Memorial Medical Center in Robbinsdale Minnesota, an Adjunct faculty member at the University of Minnesota, and faculty at University of Phoenix ONline. She received her BSN from the Univerity of Iowa, an MS and a PhD in nursing and gerontology from the Univesity of Minnesota and is certified as a CNS in gerontoloty. She has 21 years of nursing experience and has held a variety of both clinical and leadership positions in acute care settings.

Tamara Harden received a BA in psychology from the University of Kansas and is currently completing a dissertation titled, "Service Utilization among People with Cognitive Impairment: Does Living Alone Really

Make a Difference?," at the University of Massachusetts Boston. She is also completing a research fellowship funded by the National Institute of Aging at the Boston University Alzheimer's Disease Center where she continues to conduct survey and clinical research on dementia, service use, and living alone.

Joan Hyde, PhD, is co-founder and chief executive officer of Hearthstone Alzheimer Care, managing seven dementia-specific assisted living residences in the northeast since 1992. She has been involved in long-term care, senior housing policy, and health care quality research for over twenty years, formerly as senior policy analyst at the Gerontology Institute of the University of Massachusetts Boston, and currently as director of Hearthstone Alzheimer Care's research division.

Cheryl A. Lehman, RN, MSN, CRRN-A, is a clinical nurse specialist on the ACE Unit at the University of Texas Medical Branch, Galveston, Texas. She is also a doctoral candidate in preventive medicine and community health at UTMB. Professional interests include staff nurse education, measuring quality of services provided, and issues of access to healthcare services.

Jed A. Levine is executive vice president and director of programs and services at the New York City Chapter of the Alzheimer's Association. He has over 30 years experience working in Alzheimer's and dementia care. He has led efforts in the United States to include persons with these conditions in program and advocacy initiatives designed to learn directly from them about their needs.

Jean Marks, M Ed, opened the first Alzheimer's Association Chapter office in New York City and served as its program director and associate executive director until her retirement in 2000. Jean initiated and sustained the Chapter's involvement in many innovative projects to improve care for people with Alzheimer's and other dementias including the project with Cabrini Medical Center.

Mary Pat McKay, MD, MPH, is Director, Center for Injury Prevention and Control, Department of Emergency Medicine, and Associate Professor, emergency medicine and public health, George Washington University Medical Center, Washington, DC. Prior to that, she was an instructor at Harvard Medical School and an attending physician in the Department of Emergency Medicine at Brigham and Women's Hospital. Her area of expertise is motor vehicle–related injury. She was selected to serve as the Medical Fellow for the National Highway Traffic Safety Administration from 2002 to 2004, where she has been doing research specific to age-related differences in crash risk and injury severity.

Sonia Michelson, MSW, is a clinical social worker and geriatric care manager in Eastern Massachusetts, working with older adults and families who are facing the multiple challenges of aging, including changes in health and cognitive status. When families are at a distance, the geriatric care manager is actively involved in all aspects of care and functions as a liaison to other practitioners as well as to the family. Ms. Michelson is also a Lecturer at the University of Massachusetts Boston Gerontology Certificate program.

Jeffrey N. Nichols, MD, is vice president, Cabrini Eldercare Consortium and medical director of the Cabrini Center for Nursing and Rehabilitation, the St. Cabrini Nursing Home, and the Sr. Josephine Tsieu and Monsignor Terance Attridge Adult Day Health Centers. Dr. Nichols is also the assistant medical director of geriatrics and palliative care for the Cabrini Hospice. He is board certified in internal medicine and hospice and palliative care and has a certificate of added qualifications in geriatrics.

Frank W. Porell, PhD, is professor of gerontology at the John W. McCormack Graduate School of Policy Studies, University of Massachusetts Boston. His general research interests include factors affecting hospital use by community-dwelling and institutionalized elderly, geographic variations in hospital use, capitation rate risk adjustment, disability transitions among the elderly, and nursing home quality indicators.

Susan Schumacher, MS, has been a medical/surgical/geriatrics advanced practice nurse for over 10 years. Currently she coordinates the *TWICE (Together We're Improving Care for Elders) Program* at North Memorial Medical Center, developing systems to address specific needs for the geriatric population and providing education for interdisciplinary staff. Ms. Schumacher serves as a consultant for staff with patients experiencing delirium and/or dementia, as well as other complex medical or surgical needs.

Susan Tyler, RN, MSN, APRN-BC, is the administrative director for geriatric services at the University of Texas Medical Branch, Galveston, Texas. She is responsible for the acute inpatient (ACE) hospital unit, the outpatient clinical services, and for community outreach and health promotion services. Ms. Tyler has a professional interest in incontinence management in the aging population, and runs the incontinence clinic in the geriatrics clinic at UTMB.

Meredith Wallace, PhD, APRN, is an assistant professor at Fairfield University in Connecticut. She received her B.S.N. degree *magna cum laude* at Boston University, and earned an MSN in medical-surgical nursing with a specialty in geriatrics from Yale University, and a PhD in nursing research and theory development at New York University. During her time at NYU she was awarded a predoctoral fellowship at the Hartford Institute for Geriatric Nursing. In this capacity, she became the original author and editor of *Try This: Best Practices in Geriatric Nursing series.*

Cora Zembrzuski, PhD, RN, is a Building Academic Geriatric Nursing Capacity Scholar, supported by the American Academy of Nursing and the Hartford Foundation. She is an ANCC clinical specialist in gerontological nursing and a doctoral candidate at New York University. She has published in the area of dementia and hydration in older adults in the nursing home and has presented at national and regional conferences in the field of geriatrics and Alzheimer's disease.

Preface

This book is intended to bring attention to the issue of hospital care for patients with dementia. We have attempted to present a balance of what is known in the research literature and what has been experienced in practice in order to define the gaps that must be addressed. Emerging examples of best practice are also shared. This is not a book that argues the merit of treating the acute care needs of the person with dementia in the hospital versus the long-term care setting. While that is an important discussion to have, we start by acknowledging that many persons with dementia are being treated in hospital settings and probably will continue to be treated there.

The book is organized in four parts. In Part One, we provide background and discuss the significance of the issue. In Part Two, four unique perspectives are shared: the assisted living manager, the geriatric social worker, the emergency department doctor, and the person with dementia who lives alone in the community. In Part Three, we highlight four models of care implemented in hospital settings that are sensitive to the acute care needs of patients with dementia and have found creative ways to provide for those needs. In Part Four, we highlight strategies for different stakeholders in the quest to provide good dementia care in the hospital setting. Finally, we conclude by drawing some implications for policy and practice.

Fundamentally, we hope that this collection of ideas will stimulate discussion and lead to action steps—small or large—that will improve the experiences persons with dementia currently encounter in the acute care setting.

Our book is written for hospital administrators, nurses, social workers, physicians, gerontologists, psychologists, and students-in-training in all these fields. We hope the book is valuable for all advocates for better care for persons with dementia and their families.

Foreword

Eric G. Tangalos, M.D.
Mayo Clinic College of Medicine

The seeds for this book were planted more than five years ago. A group of Alzheimer's Association national board members and national and chapter staff realized the significant limitations Alzheimer's patients and their families were experiencing during acute hospital stays. To stimulate a better understanding of these issues, an Acute Care Task Force was formed, a literature search was done, and "thought leaders" were brought together to create a program initiative that would better address the problem.

Unlike Alzheimer's Association research initiatives, this program initiative received no funding from the Medical Science Advisory Council. The $70,000 set aside for an RFP came from the Association's Program Services Division. Ultimately, one hospital was chosen from sixty grant submissions to improve acute care while partnering with its local chapter of the Alzheimer's Association.

Nina Silverstein was one of those thought leaders to join us in 1999 to help the Association illuminate the problems of acute care for Alzheimer's patients. Having surveyed the landscape, she and Katie Maslow elected to take on the task of codifying the issues to bring much needed attention to the problem. This book is another outcome of that Acute Care Initiative, an educational tool in the fight against Alzheimer"s disease.

The book is divided into four parts. It covers the waterfront of acute care for persons with dementia. It focuses on hospital care primarily, but the topic ranges remarkably into the environment that brings patients to the hospital and supports them once they get out. In Part One, authors appropriately ask, "Are there dementia-friendly hospitals out there right now?" Benchmark opportunities are shared. Throughout the entire book, the editors have selected a format for storytelling. Many of us believe that the care of the elderly is really about understanding their stories, and this book is put together with very practical and experiential parables. The editors ask not only how has it been done, but how it should be done and conclude that care must improve in hospital settings.

In Part Two, individual authors go on to share perspectives on the hospital experience for persons with dementia, oftentimes through the patient's or caregiver's eyes. From the vantage point of assisted living, we see the hospital as a dangerous and risky place with not much information going in or coming out. The patient experience is also taken to the emergency room where we are treated to an in-depth analysis of the difficulties at this location. There is also the sharing of the inpatient experience from those trying to care for isolated adults with Alzheimer's disease.

Part Three shows us some promise in the care of hospitalized patients with dementia. The initiative in Oregon, which received funding from the Alzheimer's Association, is featured. Other promising models of care are also discussed.

Finally, Part Four discusses strategies for making a difference and features good nursing care for hospitalized older adults. The *Try This* series developed by the Hartford Institute for Geriatric Nursing and the Alzheimer's Association is described. *Try This* is an outstanding approach that is both simple and comprehensive. A number of topics are discussed and reviewed in detail, including avoiding restraints and pain assessment for persons with dementia.

The Alzheimer's Association New York City Chapter has been on the forefront of improving acute care. Through the Cabrini project, advocates were instrumental in demonstrating a hospital-based program that was collaborative within the city. The project also received funding from a charitable foundation and has done great work in preparing the way. It is an appropriate end to a comprehensive story that will hopefully begin a new era of care for the acutely ill patient with Alzheimer's disease.

The acute care hospital experience may be the most devastating transition patients with Alzheimer's disease or other dementias ever face. With deficits in cognition, function, and behavior all at play, negotiating an acute illness with hospitalization can be overwhelming. The risk of delirium and its antecedent morbidity in dementia patients is increased. The age burden and illness burden of our Alzheimer's patients make them vulnerable to elective as well as emergency procedures. We do get an honest look at the difficulties encountered with hospital cultures, administrations, and incentives.

Hospitals are built to provide acute care to cognitively intact individuals. The same safeguards that apply in nursing homes to protect their residents may not be a part of the hospital routine. Protecting frail or vulnerable elderly includes addressing issues of food and nutrition, hydration, toileting, and restraints. A hospitalization that neglects these issues is a life-changing event, and neither patients nor their families or caregivers ever make a full recovery. Now it is time for a change in culture, focus, and care.

Acknowledgments

We thank the many contributing authors who shared their perspectives and helped us give visibility to the critical issues in providing care for persons with dementia who are hospitalized. In developing this book, we tested ideas through offering several symposia at professional meetings, including those of the Gerontological Society of America, the American Society on Aging, the Annual Clinical Updates Conference of the Nurses Improving Care for Health System Elders (NICHE) program at New York University, the Boston Alzheimer's Symposium, and the Alzheimer's Association Annual Education Conference. Discussion generated by each of these presentations underscored the widespread concern among social and health care professionals about the lack of recognition of dementia and the need to include that recognition in the design of the hospital environment and in the determination of care plans.

The Gerontology Institute and the College of Public and Community Service at the University of Massachusetts Boston supported author Silverstein's initial exploration into this topic with her students by providing resources under the auspices of the undergraduate gerontology program and certificate in Gerontological Social Policy. Robert Geary, Managing Editor, Gerontology Institute, provided editorial assistance.

The Alzheimer's Association provided support through its *Acute Care Initiative* that enabled Silverstein and Maslow to collaborate on several projects related to improving care for hospitalized patients with dementia. Dr. Eric Tangalos, whose foreword introduces our effort, chaired that initiative.

For their patience, understanding, and continued support, special thanks to our families: Irwin, Ilana and Julie Silverstein; Surrie and Edward Melnick; and Harvey Eisen.

Introduction

Nina M. Silverstein and Katie Maslow

HOW THE IDEA FOR OUR BOOK DEVELOPED

We would like to share with the reader why and how this topic—hospital care for people with dementia—became an important area for us to explore. For Nina, the observations of a graduate student resonated with her until she found the opportunity to delve further into the realities encountered by that student. Katie's work on an initiative of the Alzheimer's Association to improve hospital care for people with dementia stimulated her interest in this generally understudied aspect of dementia care.

Terri Salmons Tobin, Ph.D., was Nina's graduate research assistant from 1994 to 1996 during which time they completed a study on wandering behavior among persons with dementia who were registered in the Alzheimer's Association *Safe Return*™ program. They interviewed over 500 caregivers of registered persons about their experiences with wandering behavior.[1] Shortly after their study ended, they received a call from a caregiver seeking information. The caregiver asked if there was a graduate student who might be interested in being provided with housing in exchange for providing respite care for her husband who was diagnosed with dementia. Terri enthusiastically replied that she herself was interested. In essence, Terri became a "walking buddy." That relationship lasted for one and a half years until the time that the husband was institutionalized.

One of Terri's early experiences as a respite care provider found her not at the couple's residence but at the emergency department in a major Boston hospital. The husband had an ear infection that was not responding well to at-home treatment by the visiting nurse. Mrs. S called Terri and asked her to meet the couple in the emergency department.

Terri later described a very crowded waiting room setting where Mr. S. was very agitated and wanted to leave repeatedly. It seemed to

---

[1]That study later became the basis for Terri's doctoral thesis. Salmons Tobin, T. (1999). *Wandering, getting lost, and Alzheimer's disease: Influences on precautions taken and levels of supervision provided by caregivers.* Unpublished doctoral thesis. University of Massachusetts Boston, MA. The study was also the basis for their co-authored book (with G. Flaherty) titled *Dementia and Wandering Behavior: Concern for the Lost Elder* (Springer).

take forever before he was seen by the emergency department physician and then needed to wait again in the general admissions waiting room until a room was available for him to be admitted to the hospital. Terri also described the amount of paperwork necessary for being seen in the emergency department and then later to be admitted to the hospital. There was no way that Mr. S. would have been able to complete the information on his own. Moreover, Mrs. S. would not have been able to complete the paperwork on her own without the reassurance that Terri was attending to the needs of Mr. S.

Once Mr. S. was settled into his room, removing his clothing to put on a hospital gown did not go smoothly—he could not understand who the hospital personnel were and why they were taking his clothes. The IV in his arm also presented a problem; he kept trying to remove it.

Next Terri encountered some examples where hospital regulations and good dementia care seemed to be in conflict. For example, Terri wanted to close the door to minimize the noise and distractions in the hallway as well as to reduce Mr. S.'s temptation to exit. Terri was asked not to close the door.

Later, Terri wanted to remove the food tray that seemed to be upsetting Mr. S. after he had eaten. She tried to move it to the hallway outside of the room; she quickly learned that that was not allowed and that she would have to wait for the hospital employee whose job it was to remove trays. There were several other incidences concerning food: the hospital employee brought the tray, with all of the individual covered items, and left it on the table; however, Mr. S., had no idea that food was under the covered plates. He was also incapable of removing the lids properly. Once he had finished, he repeatedly wanted to clean up—the dirty dishes seemed to trigger his restless behavior.

There were also incidences involving the bathroom. While most patients do not need a tour of a hospital room and specifically to be shown the location of the bathroom, Mr. S. did need such an orientation. He had no idea what was behind each door—Was it a bathroom or a closet?

He repeatedly wanted to leave his room and join the activity in the hallway. When Terri walked with him, he would try to go into other patients' rooms and had to be redirected.

It was helpful that Mr. S. was in a private room that minimized his distraction to other patients or their distraction to him. Moreover, his room was near the nurse's station so he could easily be seen in the event that he wandered off unsupervised.

It was quickly apparent that Mr. S. would need someone to stay with him overnight. Unless the family was able to pay for a private duty nurse, no other option was available through the hospital. Terri rotated shifts with Mrs. S. and their daughter until Mr. S. was discharged.

EXPLORING THE TOPIC FURTHER

In fall 1999 and spring 2000, Nina led a two-semester seminar for undergraduate gerontology majors and advanced certificate students in Gerontological Social Policy at the University of Massachusetts Boston, College of Public and Community Service (CPCS). The title of the seminar was, *How Dementia-Friendly are Acute Care Hospital Stays in Massachusetts?* CPCS is a competency-based college. In the first semester, students demonstrated two competencies: *Understanding Gerontological Social Policy* and *History of a Social Policy in Aging* by learning about Alzheimer's disease and caring for hospitalized elders. During the second semester, the students[2] conducted a research project and interviewed directors of patient care (or their equivalents) in thirty-three acute care hospitals in Massachusetts to demonstrate the competencies: *Working on a Gerontological Social Issue* and *Influencing Policy-Making*. (For more information on CPCS and competency-based education, visit www.cpcs.umb.edu). The purpose of the research project was to gather data on current practices and planned changes in the care of patients with dementia, and on perceptions about the major challenges faced in providing such care. Results of the research project are described in Chapter 2.

ALZHEIMER'S ASSOCIATION INITIATIVE ON IMPROVING HOSPITAL CARE FOR PEOPLE WITH DEMENTIA

Meanwhile, in late 1999, Katie and other Alzheimer's Association staff members had begun to work on the Association's new initiative on improving hospital care for people with dementia. The initiative was stimulated by anecdotal reports from Alzheimer's Association chapters across the country about difficult and frustrating hospital experiences encountered by individuals with dementia. Family caregivers told chapters about the same kinds of problems Terri faced as she tried to take care of Mr. S in the emergency department and hospital. The Association's National Board approved the new initiative and the allocation of Association funds for a pilot demonstration project to test approaches for improving hospital care for people with dementia.

---

[2]The following former students are acknowledged for their contribution to this project: K. Goldberg, K. Greenan, P. Hogan, U. Kabba, M. Lojek, M. MacDonald, J. MacNeill, D. Pohotsky, J. Toomey, and J. Weistrop. In addition, then doctoral candidate, L. Bruner-Canhoto also contributed to the data analysis.

Alzheimer's Association staff collected information, including research articles, about the topic. Staff also contacted knowledgeable physicians, nurses, and other health care professionals across the country to learn more about the problems in hospital care for people with dementia and any approaches that were being tested to improve care. The Association's New York City Chapter had already begun working with Cabrini Medical Center on the development of an acute care unit for hospital patients with dementia.[3] A visit to that unit in early 2000 helped staff from the Association's national office understand what was possible in terms of high quality care for hospital patients with dementia.

In September 2000, the Alzheimer's Association convened an advisory panel to identify the most important issues to be addressed in improving hospital care for people with dementia, and to establish goals for the pilot demonstration project, and set criteria for selecting a site for the project.[4] Based on the recommendations of the advisory panel, the Association issued a request for letters of intent for the pilot demonstration project. Advisory panel members and Association staff wondered what kind of response there would be and were pleased and amazed when letters of intent were received from more than sixty hospitals, including hospitals of all sizes and from all across the country. One requirement for the demonstration project was a working partnership between the hospital and its local Alzheimer's Association chapter. Association chapters were also pleased and amazed when important hospitals in their communities contacted them to partner on a proposal for the pilot demonstration project.

With great difficulty, the advisory panel and staff selected ten of the sixty letters of intent and asked those hospitals to submit a full proposal. Then, with even greater difficulty, the panel and staff chose one hospital, Providence Milwaukie Hospital in Oregon, to receive the grant. The panel and staff wished that additional funds were available to support at least the ten projects for which full proposals were submitted. Provi-

---

[3]The Cabrini Acute Care Unit is described in Chapter 11 of this book. The New York City Chapter's role in the project is described in Chapter 13.

[4]The panel was chaired by Eric G. Tangalos, MD, of the Mayo Clinic. Dr. Tangalos is also a member of the National Board of the Alzheimer's Association. The following individuals were members of the advisory panel: Kara Albisu, MSW; Harrison Bloom, MD; Mary Bouche; Uriel Cohen, MArch, ArchD; Geri Hall, RN, PhD; Paul Harrington, MSW; Sheldon Lewin, LCSW; Katie Maslow, MSW; Mary Naylor, RN, PhD; Jeffrey Nichols, MD; Judy Riggs; Nina M. Silverstein, PhD; Danita Vetter, MA, CGC; and Robert M. Wachter, MD, FACP.

dence Milwaukie Hospital and the Oregon Trails Chapter conducted their pilot demonstration project from 2001 to 2003.[5]

Among the ten hospitals that were asked for a full proposal for the pilot demonstration project, three hospitals, including Providence Milwaukie Hospital, described themselves as "NICHE" hospitals. Association staff members wondered about "NICHE" and quickly learned that "Nurses Improving Care for Health System Elders" (NICHE) was a project of John A. Hartford Institute for Geriatric Nursing at New York University. The directors of the Hartford Institute expressed strong interest in improving hospital care for people with dementia, and a partnership was created between the Institute and the Alzheimer's Association for this purpose. One result of this partnership has been *Try This: Best Practices in Nursing Care for Hospitalized Older Adults with Dementia*, a series of brief documents intended to help hospital nurses understand and respond to common problems in dementia care.[6]

Our initial work on the topic of hospital care for people with Alzheimer's disease and other dementias increased our concerns about the difficult experiences confronted by hospital patients with these conditions and their families. It also introduced us to other advocates, researchers, and health care and social service professionals—both inside and outside hospitals—who share our concerns and have begun to work in various ways to improve the current reality. Our book assembles information and ideas intended to support these efforts. We hope it illuminates the problem and increases awareness of promising strategies for change. Most importantly, we hope it motivates others to seek ways to make a difference in this understudied but very difficult and critical aspect of the care continuum for people with Alzheimer's and other dementias.

---

[5]The project conducted by Providence Milwaukie Hospital and the Oregon Trails Chapter is described in Chapter 8 of this book.
[6]The *Try This* series is described in Chapter 12 of this book.

PART I

Background and Significance

CHAPTER ONE

How Many People with Dementia Are Hospitalized?

Katie Maslow

There are no generally accepted figures for the number or proportion of people with Alzheimer's disease and other dementias who are hospitalized. Hospital care has received far less attention from researchers than other types and settings of care for people with these conditions. Some researchers and clinicians believe that people with dementia are physically healthier than other elderly people and therefore less likely to be hospitalized. Some believe that other types and settings of care are more central to the overall experience of a person with dementia and therefore more important topics for research. In addition, many hospital patients who have dementia do not have a dementia diagnosis in their hospital records. As a result, it is difficult to obtain the data needed to develop credible figures on the number who are hospitalized.

This chapter presents the available information about the number and proportion of people with dementia who are hospitalized each year. It summarizes findings from studies that compare hospitalization rates for people with and without dementia and discusses factors that have been shown to affect these rates. Because usual practices for hospitalization differ greatly in different countries, only findings from studies conducted in the United States are discussed in the chapter.

The question of how many people with dementia are hospitalized can be addressed from three perspectives: (1) the population or societal perspective; (2) the perspective of the person, his or her family, and care providers outside the hospital; and (3) the perspective of the hospital. From the population or societal perspective, the most important answers to the question pertain to the total number and cost of hospital stays for people with dementia. From the perspective of the person, his or her family, and nonhospital care providers, the most important answer pertains to the proportion of people with dementia who have one or more hospitalizations in a given time period. From the hospital perspective, the most important answers pertain to the number of patients with dementia who are in the hospital at any given time or over time and the proportion of all hospital patients who have dementia. All three perspectives are represented in the following chapters, and all three are critical for understanding the problems in hospital care for people with dementia and devising solutions for those problems.

As noted above, many hospital patients with dementia do not have a dementia diagnosis in their hospital records. Probably as many as half of all people with dementia have never received a formal diagnosis, and even those who have been diagnosed may not have their diagnosis noted in their hospital admission or discharge records. Hospital staff may or may not recognize dementia in patients whose records contain nothing about their cognitive deficits. Problems associated with the lack of recognition of dementia in hospital patients are discussed in every chapter of this book. Better procedures for the recognition and documentation of dementia are essential for improved care.

Better procedures for recognition and documentation of dementia are also essential for the development of accurate information about the number and proportion of people with dementia who are hospitalized and the proportion of hospital patients who have dementia. Even without this information, however, it is clear that hospitalization is a common occurrence for people with dementia. The chapter concludes that in 2000, there were as many as 3.2 million hospital stays in the United States that involved a person with dementia; about one-third of people with dementia are hospitalized each year, some more than once; and about one-fourth of elderly hospital patients have dementia. These substantial figures provide ample evidence that hospital care is an important issue for future dementia research. The figures also mean that many people with dementia, families, and hospital and non-hospital care providers are affected by the problems described in other chapters of this book.

NUMBER AND COST OF HOSPITAL STAYS
FOR PEOPLE WITH DEMENTIA

The great majority of people with dementia are age 65 and over and eligible for Medicare. Thus, Medicare data are useful for estimating the number and cost of hospital stays for people with dementia. Information about the number and cost of hospital stays addresses the question, How many people with dementia are hospitalized? from a population or societal perspective.

Medicare data for a nationally representative sample of beneficiaries aged 65+ show that in 2000, those with dementia had 1,091 hospital stays per 1,000 beneficiaries (see Table 1.1). These data are based on Medicare claims for a 5% random sample of Medicare fee-for-service beneficiaries that is generated each year by the Centers for Medicare and Medicaid Services (CMS), the federal government agency that administers Medicare.[1] The data show the average number of hospital stays per thousand beneficiaries and include beneficiaries who had no hospital stays and beneficiaries who had one or more hospital stays in the year. For this analysis, beneficiaries are considered to have dementia if they had at least one Medicare claim during the year that included a diagnostic code for Alzheimer's disease or another dementia.[2]

In 2000, the Medicare 5% sample represented about 25 million elderly beneficiaries, including 2.2 million beneficiaries with dementia. With 2.2 million beneficiaries and 1,091 hospital stays per thousand beneficiaries, there would have been about 2.4 million hospital stays involving a person with dementia in 2000.

No comparable government data are available for the approximately 10 million elderly beneficiaries who are not represented in the 5% sample, e.g., beneficiaries enrolled in Medicare managed care (HMOs) and those who receive medical care through the Department of Veterans Affairs (VA). If the proportion of beneficiaries with dementia were the same for these other beneficiaries as for fee-for-service beneficiaries (9%), and if the number of hospital stays per thousand were the same (1,091 per 1,000), there would have been almost one million additional hospital stays involving a person with dementia in 2000, for a total of 3.2 million hospital stays.

The 3.2 million figure does not imply that dementia caused the hospital stays, only that the stays involved a person with dementia. Moreover, the 3.2 million figure is an estimate, and the true number could be lower or higher. It could be lower if some of the fee-for-service beneficiaries with hospital stays in 2000 had a Medicare claim with a diagnostic

---

[1]The claims included in the analysis reported here are for people aged 65+ who were enrolled in regular, fee-for-service Medicare and had both Part A and Part B coverage for the full year (or while they were alive).

[2]The diagnostic codes used to identify beneficiaries with Alzheimer's disease and other dementias are ICD-9 codes 290, 294, and 331. These codes could appear on Medicare claims for hospital care, physician visits, home health care, or any other Medicare-covered service.

TABLE 1.1 Hospitalizations per 1,000 Medicare Beneficiaries aged 65+ and Average Hospital Costs per Beneficiary With and Without Dementia and Coexisting Medical Conditions, 2000

Medicare fee-for-service beneficiaries aged 65+	Number of beneficiaries in the 5% sample	Average hospital stays per 1,000 beneficiaries	Average hospital costs per beneficiary ($)
All beneficiaries aged 65+	1,246,427	387	2,640
All beneficiaries with no dementia	1,134,642	318	2,204
All beneficiaries with dementia	111,785	1,091	7,074
With diabetes			
All with diabetes, no dementia + any/none[1]	190,215	587	4,207
All with diabetes + dementia + any/none	25,276	1,589	10,943
With CHF[2]			
All with CHF, no dementia + any/none	114,258	1,259	9,441
All with CHF + dementia + any/none	30,945	1,901	13,178
With COPD[3]			
All with COPD, no dementia + any/none	107,782	1,054	7,580
All with COPD + dementia + any/none	19,370	2,022	13,980

[1]Any/none = With or without any other chronic condition.

[2]CHF = Congestive heart failure.

[3] COPD = Chronic obstructive pulmonary disease, including emphysema.

Source: U.S. Centers for Medicare and Medicaid (CMS), 5% national random sample of fee-for-service Medicare claims for 2000.

code for dementia but really did not have dementia. The true number could also be lower if the proportion of people with dementia and/or the number of hospital stays per thousand were lower in Medicare HMOs or VA than in fee-for-service Medicare. The true number could be higher if some fee-for-service beneficiaries with dementia had one or more hospital stays but did not have a Medicare claim in 2000 with diagnostic code for dementia. Despite these caveats, the 3.2 million figure is useful as a ballpark estimate of the number of hospital stays involving a person with dementia in 2000.

Before turning to other types and sources of information, several additional findings from the Medicare 5% sample should be noted. The first finding pertains to the effect of coexisting medical conditions on the number of hospital stays. Many people with dementia also have other, serious medical conditions (Bynum, Rabins, Weller, Niefeld, Anderson, & Wu, 2004; Hill, Futterman, Duttagupta, Mastey, Lloyd, & Fillit, 2002; Maslow, 2004). Data from the Medicare 5% sample show, for example, that in 2000, 23% of elderly fee-for-service Medicare beneficiaries with dementia also had diabetes; 28% also had congestive heart failure (CHF); and 17% also had chronic obstructive pulmonary disease (COPD) (Alzheimer's Association, 2003).

One might guess that coexisting medical conditions account for the high number of hospital stays per thousand for people with dementia. That appears to be true in the Medicare 5% sample, but it is not the whole story. In 2000, beneficiaries with diabetes plus dementia had a higher number of hospital stays per thousand than the average for all beneficiaries with dementia (1,589 vs. 1,091 hospital stays per 1,000) (see Table 1.1). In addition, however, beneficiaries with diabetes plus dementia had a higher number of hospital stays per thousand than the average for beneficiaries with diabetes but no dementia (1,589 vs. 587 hospital stays per 1,000). Thus, in this sample at least, coexisting diabetes increased the number of hospital stays for beneficiaries with dementia, and conversely, coexisting dementia increased the number of hospital stays for beneficiaries with diabetes. The same effect can be seen for CHF and COPD (see Table 1.1).

The second finding to be noted from the Medicare 5% sample pertains to the effect of age on the number of hospital stays. Among Medicare beneficiaries aged 65+, those with dementia are older, on average, than other beneficiaries. In 2000, for example, 38% of beneficiaries aged 65+ with dementia were aged 85+, compared with only 11% of other beneficiaries. One might guess that the older average age of beneficiaries with dementia accounts for their high number of hospital stays. That does not appear to be true in this sample. As shown in Table 1.2, the number of hospital stays per thousand for beneficiaries with dementia

TABLE 1.2 Hospitalizations per 1,000 Medicare Beneficiaries and Average Hospital Costs per Beneficiary with Dementia, 2000

Medicare fee-for-service beneficiaries	Number of beneficiaries in the 5% sample	Average hospital stays per 1,000 beneficiaries	Average hospital costs per beneficiary ($)
Age 65–74			
All beneficiaries	623,357	295	2,151
All with no dementia	603,321	262	1,912
All with dementia	20,036	1,268	9,327
Age 75–84			
All beneficiaries	458,553	443	3,036
All with no dementia	409,262	362	2,511
All with dementia	49,291	1,117	7,388
Age 85+			
All beneficiaries	164,517	581	3,394
All with no dementia	122,059	442	2,611
All with dementia	42,458	978	5,646

[1]Any/none = With or without any other chronic condition.

Source: U.S. Centers for Medicare and Medicaid (CMS), 5% national random sample of fee-for-service Medicare claims for 2000.

actually decreases with age, from 1,268 stays per 1,000 for those aged 65–74, to 1,117 stays per 1,000 for those aged 75–84, and 978 stays per 1,000 for those aged 85+.

Data from the Medicare 5% sample can be used to compare the number of hospital stays per thousand for Medicare beneficiaries with dementia and other Medicare beneficiaries. Data for 2000 show that beneficiaries with dementia had 3.4 times more hospital stays than other beneficiaries (1,091 vs. 381 hospital stays per 1,000 beneficiaries) (see Table 1.1). Data from the same source show that in 1999, elderly Medicare beneficiaries with dementia had 3.8 times more hospital stays per thousand than other Medicare beneficiaries (Bynum et al., 2004).

The difference in hospital stays per thousand is highest for beneficiaries aged 65–74 and decreases in older age groups. In the age group 65–74, beneficiaries with dementia had almost five times more hospital stays than other beneficiaries (1,268 vs. 262 hospital stays per 1,000). In contrast, in the age group 75–84, beneficiaries with dementia had three times more hospital stays (1,117 vs. 362 stays per 1,000), and in the age group 85+, those with dementia had only two times more hospital stays (978 vs. 442 stays per 1,000).

Medicare costs for hospital care are consistent with the number of hospital stays. The data show that in 2000, hospital care for beneficiaries with dementia cost Medicare 3.3 times more than hospital care for beneficiaries without dementia ($7,074 vs. $2,204 per sampled beneficiary) (see Table 1.1). Coexisting diabetes, CHF, and COPD increased Medicare hospital costs for those with dementia, and conversely, dementia increased Medicare hospital costs for those with diabetes, CHF, and COPD. The highest Medicare hospital costs were for younger beneficiaries ($9,327 for those aged 65–74 vs. $5,646 for those aged 85+), and the difference in hospital costs for beneficiaries with and without dementia was greater for those aged 65–74 than for those aged 85+ (see Table 1.2).

PROPORTION OF PEOPLE WITH DEMENTIA WHO ARE HOSPITALIZED

Information about the proportion of people with dementia who are hospitalized addresses the question, How many people with dementia are hospitalized? from the perspective of the person with dementia, his or her family, and other nonhospital care providers, such as nursing homes, assisted living facilities, and geriatric care managers. The important issue from this perspective is the likelihood that a person with dementia will be hospitalized in a given period of time.

From 1990 to 2004, at least ten studies were published that reported on the proportion of people with dementia who were hospitalized in the United States in a given period of time. The samples for these studies differ in many ways, including how people with dementias were identified, their insurance status (e.g., Medicare fee-for-service, Medicare managed care (HMOs), Medicaid), their age, and whether they lived at home or in a nursing home.

Five of the ten studies used a brief mental status test to identify people with dementia and included only people who lived at home. Of the five studies:

- One study found that 31% of people with dementia aged 70+ were hospitalized at least once in a one-year period (Walsh, Wu, Mitchell, & Berkmann, 2003).
- Three studies found that 19 to 33% of people aged 65+ with mild dementia and 29 to 38% of those with moderate or severe dementia were hospitalized at least once in a one-year period (Binder & Robins, 1990; Callahan, Hendrie, & Tierney, 1995; Kasper, 1995).

- One study found that 19% of people aged 65+ were hospitalized at least once in a six-month period (Ganguli, Seaberg, Belle, Fischer, & Kuller, 1993).

Another four studies used diagnostic information to identify people with dementia:

- Two of these studies focused on Medicaid recipients, including recipients aged 50+ in Georgia and recipients aged 60+ in California (Martin, Ricci, Kotzan, Lang, & Menzin, 2000; Menzin, Lang, Friedman, Neumann, & Cummings, 1999). Both studies included a high proportion of nursing home residents (87% and 65%, respectively). In the Georgia sample, 30% of the people with dementia were hospitalized at least once in a one-year period, compared with only 14% in the California sample.
- One study of people aged 65+ with a diagnosis of dementia found that 76% were hospitalized at least once in a four-year period (Leibson, Owens, O'Brien, Waring, Tangalos, & Hanson, et al.
- One study of people aged 65+ with a diagnosis of dementia in a Medicare HMO found that 40% were hospitalized at least once in a one-year period (Richards, Shepherd, Crismon, Snyder, & Jermain, 2000).

The last of the ten studies of this type (Fillenbaum, Heyman, Peterson, Pieper, & Weiman, 2001) found that among people aged 65+ with a diagnosis of dementia, the proportion that was hospitalized differed, depending on stage of dementia and whether the people with dementia lived at home or in a nursing home. For those who lived at home, the proportion hospitalized at least once in a one-year period *increased* with stage of dementia from 13% of those in the earliest stage to 29% of those in the latest stage. In contrast, among those who lived in a nursing home, the proportion hospitalized at least once in a one-year period *decreased* with stage of dementia, from 27% of those in the earliest stage to 15% of those in the latest stage.

Eight of the ten studies above provide data for a 1-year period. The results of these eight studies support a tentative conclusion that, on average, about one-third of people with dementia are hospitalized at least once in a one-year period. It is not possible to determine whether the results of the two studies that provide data for a six-month and four-year period (Ganguli et al., 1993; Liebson et al., 1999) are consistent with this conclusion. Exceptions to the conclusion are the smaller proportions reported for California Medicaid recipients (14%), people with mild or early stage of dementia who live at home (13–19%), and people with late-stage dementia who live in nursing homes (15%).

Five of the ten studies report the average number of hospitalizations for people with dementia who had at least one hospitalization in a one-year period. The reported average is 1.5 to 2 hospitalizations a year, with a range of 1 to 8 hospitalizations per person (Callahan et al., 1995; Fillenbaum, et al., 2001; Liebson et al., 1999; Richards et al., 2000; Walsh et al., 2003).

As with the figure on hospital stays discussed in the preceding section, the tentative conclusion that about one-third of people with dementia are hospitalized in a year does not imply that dementia caused the hospitalizations. It only indicates that these hospitalizations involved a person with dementia.

COMPARING HOSPITALIZATION RATES AND COSTS FOR PEOPLE WITH AND WITHOUT DEMENTIA

From 1990 to 2004, at least twenty-six studies were published that compared hospitalization rates for people with and without dementia in U.S. samples consisting of people who lived at home only or people who lived at home and people who lived in nursing homes.[3] Some of the findings summarized in this section are based on information about hospitalization rates, including number of hospital stays and the proportion of people with and without dementia who are hospitalized in a given period of time. Other findings are based on information about the cost of hospital stays for people with and without dementia. Information about hospitalization rates and costs is combined for purposes of comparison, and statistical significance is noted.

- Eleven of the twenty-six studies had statistically significant findings showing higher hospitalization rates or costs for people with dementia regardless of adjustments for any other factors considered in the study; four of these studies used samples of Medicare fee-for-service beneficiaries aged 65+ (Bynum et al., 2004; Fillenbaum, Heyman, Peterson, Pieper, & Weiman, 2000; Taylor & Sloan, 2000; Weiner, Powe, Weller, Shaffer, & Anderson, 1998); four of the studies used samples of Medicare managed care beneficiaries aged 65+ (Gutterman, Markowitz, Lewis, &

[3]Some of the same studies were cited in the preceding sections with respect to hospitalization rates for people with dementia only.

Fillit;[4] Hill, Fillit, Futterman, Leaderer, & Shah, 2004; Hill et al., 2002; Richards et al., 2000); and three of the studies used samples of Medicaid recipients, including people as young as aged 50 (Martin et al., 2000; Menzin et al., 1999; Weiler, Lubben, & Chi, 1991).

- Four of the twenty-six studies had statistically significant findings showing higher hospitalization rates for people with dementia regardless of adjustments for any other factors considered in the study, but the higher rates were only for those with moderate or severe dementia, not those with mild dementia (Albert, Costa, Merchant, Small, Jenders, & Stern, 1999; Binder & Robins, 1990; Callahan et al., 1995; Kasper, 1995).

- One of the twenty-six studies had statistically significant findings showing higher hospitalization costs for people with dementia admitted for hip fracture, stroke, and pneumonia, but not for people with dementia admitted for coronary heart disease or congestive heart failure (Sloan & Taylor, 2002).

- Five of the twenty-six studies had statistically significant findings showing higher hospitalization rates or costs for people with dementia before adjustment for other factors, but rates or costs were no longer higher after the adjustments (Bloom, Chhatre, & Jayadevappa, 2004; Eaker, Mickel, Chyou, Mueller-Rizner, & Slusser, 2002; Ganguli et al., 1993; Kane & Atherly, 2000; Walsh et al., 2003).[5]

- Four of the studies found no statistically significant difference in hospitalization rates for people with and without dementia (Leibson et al., 1999; McCormick, Kukull, Van Belle, Bowen, Teri, & Larson, 1995; Welch, Walsh, & Larson,1992; Wieland et al., 2000).

- One study had statistically significant findings showing a lower hospitalization rate for people with dementia (McCormick et al., 2001).

The majority of these twenty-six studies found a statistically significant relationship between dementia and higher hospitalization rates and costs, but many factors affected this relationship, and adjustments based on some of the factors caused the relationship to disappear completely

---

[4]The sample for this study also included beneficiaries aged 60–64.

[5]Factors for which adjustments were made in one or more of these studies include age, gender, marital status, race, income, education, insurance status, severity of cognitive impairment, coexisting medical conditions, self-rated health, functional limitations, smoking, alcohol intake, use of other health care services, proxy status, and follow-back time.

or lose statistical significance. Moreover, five of the twenty-six studies found no statistically significant relationship between dementia and hospitalization rates, and one study found a negative relationship.

Given these findings and the many differences in the study samples and procedures, it is not possible to conclude that people with dementia have higher hospitalization rates or costs without regard for other factors. Nor is it possible to conclude that there is no significant difference in hospitalization rates or costs for people with and without dementia or that people with dementia have lower hospitalization rates or costs. Further research and analysis are needed to clarify this relationship.

FACTORS THAT AFFECT HOSPITALIZATION RATES AND COSTS FOR PEOPLE WITH DEMENTIA

Many factors have been shown to affect hospitalization rates and costs for people with dementia. Perhaps the most important and interesting of these factors is whether the person with dementia lives at home or in a nursing home. The study by Kane and Atherly (2000) cited earlier found that Medicare costs for hospital care were much higher for elderly beneficiaries with dementia who lived at home than for those who lived in a nursing home. Other studies have had the same finding (see, e.g., Rice, Fox, Max, Webber, Lindeman, & Hauck, et al., 1993). Kane and Atherly (2000) also found that among all elderly Medicare beneficiaries who lived at home, those with dementia had higher Medicare costs for hospital care; in contrast, among all elderly Medicare beneficiaries who lived in nursing homes, those with dementia had lower Medicare costs for hospital care.

Many other studies focused only on nursing home residents have found lower hospitalization rates and costs for those with dementia vs. other residents (see, e.g., Burton, German, Gruber-Baldini, Hebel, Zimmerman, & Magaziner, 2001; Carter & Porell, 2003). In Chapter 3 of this book, Carter and Porell (2005) discuss these findings and point out that although hospitalization rates are generally lower for residents with dementia, individual nursing homes vary greatly in the number and proportion of their residents that are hospitalized each year. Carter and Porell discuss facility-level and market factors associated with this variation (e.g., nonprofit vs. for-profit status, staffing ratios, and reimbursement rates) and the implications of the variation in hospitalization rates for the care and well-being of residents with dementia.

The generally low hospitalization rate for nursing home residents with dementia may help to explain the results of some studies cited earlier. In particular, two studies that found no statistically significant difference in hospitalization rates for people with and without dementia (Leibson et al., 1999; Welch et al., 1992) used samples in which more than 60% of sample members with dementia lived in a nursing home at some point in the study.

In addition to whether the person with dementia lives at home or in a nursing home, several other patient-level factors have been shown to affect hospitalization rates and costs for people with dementia. These factors include:

- *Type of dementia:* two studies that compared hospitalization rates and costs for people with Alzheimer's disease vs. other dementias found higher rates and costs for those with other dementias, including vascular dementia (Eaker et al., 2002; McCormick, Hardy, Kukull, Bowen, Teri, & Zitzer, et al., 2001). Hill et al. (2004) compared hospitalization rates and costs for people with Alzheimer's disease, vascular dementia, and other types of dementia, and found a much higher rate and cost for those with vascular dementia.
- *Severity and worsening of cognitive impairment:* four studies cited earlier found higher hospitalization rates for people with moderate or severe cognitive impairment vs. those with mild cognitive impairment (Albert et al., 1999; Binder & Robins, 1990; Callahan et al., 1995; Kasper, 1995); two additional studies found that people whose cognitive status worsened over one to three years, either with new onset or increasing severity, had higher hospitalization rates than people whose cognitive status was stable (Binder & Robins, 1990; Chodesh, Seeman, Keeler, Sewell, Hirsch, & Guralnik, et al., 2004).
- *Presence of psychiatric symptoms:* two studies that compared hospitalization rates for people with dementia who did and did not have psychiatric symptoms, such as depression and psychosis, found that those with psychiatric symptoms had a higher hospitalization rate (Kales, Blow, Copeland, Bingham, Kammerer, & Mellow, 1999; Kunik. Snow, Molinari, Menke, Souchek, Sullivan, & Ashton, 2003).

The patient-level factors that affect hospitalization rates and costs mean that studies conducted in samples that include people with dementia who differ on any of these factors are likely to have different findings about rates and costs. The facility-level and market factors that affect hospitalization rates and costs for nursing home residents with dementia mean that studies conducted in different nursing homes are likely to have different findings about rates and costs. Because facility-level factors change over time, hospitalization rates and costs are also likely to change for particular nursing homes. When market factors change, hospitalization rates and costs are likely to change for all nursing homes in the region affected by the change. Thus, findings about hospitalization rates and costs for people with dementia can be expected to change over time and differ in various regions of the country.

NUMBER AND PROPORTION OF HOSPITAL PATIENTS WITH DEMENTIA

Information about the number and proportion of hospital patients who have dementia addresses the question, How many people with dementia are hospitalized? from the hospital's perspective. One answer to this question can be estimated on the basis of the data on hospital stays in Table 1.1. As shown there, 1,246,427 beneficiaries aged 65+ in the 5% Medicare sample had 387 hospital stays per thousand in 2000, for a total of 482,367 hospital stays. Likewise, 111,785 beneficiaries with dementia had 1,091 hospital stays per thousand in 2000, for a total 121,957 hospital stays. A comparison of the figures for total hospital stays shows that one-fourth of all the hospital stays for beneficiaries in this nationally representative sample involved a person with dementia. From the hospital perspective, a hospital stay is the same as a patient in the hospital. Thus, in this sample at least, one-fourth of elderly hospital patients were patients with dementia.

Five studies published from 1990 to 2004 provide information about the proportion of patients who have dementia in U.S. hospitals. Four of the five studies provide data for only one hospital, and the fifth study provides data for two hospitals. In addition, the study findings vary greatly depending on the way people with dementia were identified.

At one extreme, Lyketsos, Sheppard, and Rabins, (2000) used hospital discharge records to identify patients with a diagnosis of dementia among more than 21,000 patients aged 60+ who were admitted to Johns Hopkins University Hospital from 1996 to 1997. These researchers found that only 3.9% of the patients had dementia as identified by a discharge diagnosis.

In contrast, Sands, Yaffe, Covinsky, Chren, Counsell, & Palmer, et al., (2003) used a brief mental status test to identify patients with cognitive impairment consistent with dementia among more than 2,500 patients aged 70+ who were admitted to two Ohio hospitals from 1993 to 1996. These researchers found that 42% of the patients had dementia as identified by the mental status test.

The remaining three studies, all of which focused primarily on delirium in hospital patients, found proportions of patients with dementia between these two extremes:

- A study conducted at Beth Israel Hospital in Boston identified patients who had any mention of dementia, Alzheimer's disease, or cognitive impairment in their hospital record from a sample of 291 patients aged 65+ who were admitted to medical and surgical units in the hospital from 1987 to 1989 (Murray, Levkoff, Werle, Beckett, Cleary, & Schor, et al., 1993). This study found that 20% of these patients had dementia.
- A study conducted at Yale New Haven Hospital also identified patients with any mention of dementia, Alzheimer's disease, or cognitive impairment in their hospital record in a sample of 525 patients aged 70+ who were admitted to medical units in the hospital from 1989 to 1991 (Inouye, Bogardus, Vitagliano, Desai, Williams, & Grady, et al., 2003). This study found that 28% of these patients had dementia.
- A study conducted at the University of Chicago Hospital used a brief mental status test to identify patients with dementia in a sample of 432 patients aged 65+ who were admitted to two general medical units and two surgical units in the hospital from 1989 to 1991 (Pompei, Foreman, Rudberg, Inouye, Braund, & Cassel, 1994). This study found that 37% of these patients had dementia.

Some and perhaps many patients with dementia were excluded from the samples for the three latter studies. Murray et al. (1993) excluded patients who had delirium at the time of hospital admission. Since delirium often coexists with dementia in elderly hospital patients (Elie, Cole, Primeau, & Bellavance, 1998; Fick, Agostini, & Inouye, 2002), it is likely that the exclusion of patients with delirium resulted in an undercount of patients with dementia. Inouye et al. (2003) excluded patients with severe dementia from their sample, and Pompei et al. (1994) excluded patients who were not able to provide consent because of cognitive impairment. These exclusions probably also resulted in an undercount of patients with dementia.

Given the small number of studies, the small number of hospitals represented in the studies, and the differences in the way people with dementia were identified, it is difficult to draw any conclusion about the proportion of hospital patients who have dementia. For purposes of discussion, the author tentatively estimates that at least one-fourth of elderly hospital patients have dementia. This estimate reflects the proportion of hospital patients who had dementia in the 5% Medicare sample for 2000. It is below the middle of the range of figures from the three studies in the bulleted list above (20–37%), and the exclusions from those three studies mean that the range itself is probably low. On the other hand, the tertiary care hospitals in which the three studies were conducted and the particular units that were included in the studies may have a higher proportion of elderly patients with dementia than regular community hospitals. For these and other reasons, the estimate is uncertain but still perhaps useful as a ballpark figure for the proportion of elderly hospital patients with dementia in U.S. hospitals.

CONCLUSIONS

In 2000, an estimated 3.2 million hospitalizations involved an elderly person with dementia. On average, about one-third of people with dementia are hospitalized at least once in a one-year period, and those who are hospitalized once have an average of 1.5 to 2 hospitalizations in the year. Lastly, this author estimates that across all hospitals in the United States, an average of about one-fourth of all elderly patients have dementia.

As noted throughout this chapter, these figures do not imply that the hospitalizations are caused by dementia. The importance of the figures for people with dementia, their families, and hospital and nonhospital caregivers does not require that the hospitalizations be caused by dementia, only that they involve a person with dementia. If one-third of people with dementia are hospitalized at least once a year, a very large number of individuals, their families, and other nonhospital care providers are experiencing the problems with hospital care for people with dementia that are described in other chapters of this book. Likewise, if one fourth of elderly hospital patients are people with dementia, a very large number of physicians, nurses, nurse aides, social workers, and other hospital employees across the country are coping with the problems in providing care for hospital patients with dementia that are also described in other chapters in this book.

The numbers help to frame the issue of hospital care for people with dementia. The following chapters fill in that frame with quantitative and qualitative information about problems and potential solutions. Hopefully, the product will encourage efforts by researchers, Alzheimer's advocates, and hospital administrators and employees to improve the hospital experience for people with dementia.

REFERENCES

Albert, S. M., Costa, R., Merchant, C., Small, S., Jenders, R. A., & Stern, Y. (1999). Hospitalization and Alzheimer's disease: Results from a community-based study. *Journal of Gerontology: Medical Sciences, 54A(5)*, M267–M271.

Alzheimer's Association. (2003). Alzheimer's Disease and Chronic Health Conditions: The Real Challenge for 21st Century Medicare. Available from http://www.alz.org/Advocacy/downloads/2003ChronicCareReport.pdf

Binder, E. F., & Robins, L. N. (1990). Cognitive impairment and length of hospital stay in older persons. *Journal of the American Geriatrics Society, 38(7)*, 759–766.

Bloom, B. S., Chhatre, S., & Jayadevappa, R. (2004). Cost effects of a specialized care center for people with Alzheimer's disease. *American Journal of Alzheimer's Disease and Other Dementias,19(4)*, 226–232.

Burton, L. C., German, P. S., Gruber-Baldini, A. L., Hebel, J. R., Zimmerman S., & Magaziner, J. (2001). Medical care for nursing home residents: Differences by dementia status. *Journal of the American Geriatrics Society, 49(2)*, 142–147.

Bynum, J. P. W., Rabins, P. V., Weller, W., Niefeld, M., Anderson, G. F., & Wu, A. W. (2004). The relationship between a dementia diagnosis, chronic illness, Medicare expenditures, and hospital use. *Journal of the American Geriatrics Society, 52(2)*, 187–194.

Callahan, D. M., Hendrie, H. C., & Tierney, W. M. (1995). Documentation and evaluation of cognitive impairment in elderly primary care patients. *Annals of Internal Medicine, 122(6)*, 422–429.

Carter, M. W., & Porell, F. W., (2005). Acute care for nursing home residents with Alzheimer's disease: Understanding variations in hospital care. In N. M. Silverstein & K. Maslow (Eds.), *Improving hospital care for people with dementia*. New York: Springer.

Carter, M. W., & Porell, F. W. (2003). Variations in hospitalization rates among nursing home residents: The role of facility and market attributes. *Gerontologist, 43(2)*, 175–191.

Chodesh, J., Seeman, T. E., Keeler, E., Sewall, A., Hirsch, S. H., & Guralnik, J. M., et al. (2004). Cognitive decline in high-functioning older persons is associated with an increased risk of hospitalization. *Journal of the American Geriatrics Society, 52(9)*, 1456–1462.

Eaker, E. D., Mickel, S. F., Chyou, P., Mueller-Rizner, N. J., & Slusser, J. P. (2002). Alzheimer's disease or other dementia and medical care utilization. *Annals of Epidemiology, 12(1)*, 39–45.

Elie, M., Cole, M. G., Primeau, F. J., & Bellavance, F. J. (1998). Delirium risk factors in elderly hospitalized patients. *Journal of General Internal Medicine, 13*, 204–212.

Fick, D. M., Agostini, J. V., & Inouye, S. K. (2002). Delirium superimposed on dementia: A systematic review. *Journal of the American Geriatrics Society, 50(10)*, 1723–1732.

Fillenbaum, G., Heyman, A., Peterson, B. L., Pieper, C., & Weiman, A. L. (2000). Frequency and duration of hospitalization with Alzheimer's disease based on Medicare data: CERAD XX. *Neurology, 54,* 740–743.

Fillenbaum, G., Heyman, A., Peterson, B. L., Pieper, C. F., & Weiman, A. L. (2001). Use and cost of hospitalization of patients with Alzheimer's disease by stage and living arrangement: CERAD XX. *Neurology, 56,* 201–206.

Ganguli, M., Seaberg, E., Belle, S., Fischer L., & Kuller, L. H. (1993). Cognitive impairment and the use of health services in an elderly rural population: The MoVIES Project. *Journal of the American Geriatrics Society, 41*(10), 1065–1070.

Gutterman, E.M., Markowitz, J. S., Lewis, B., & Fillit, H. (1999). Cost of Alzheimer's disease and related dementia in managed-Medicare. *Journal of the American Geriatrics Society, 47*(9), 1065–1071.

Hill, J. W., Fillit, H., Futterman, R., Leaderer, M., & Shah, S. N. (2004). *Healthcare costs of vascular dementia in community-dwelling patients.* Paper presented at the 9th International Conference on Alzheimer's Disease and Related Disorders, July 17–22, 2004.

Hill, J. W., Futterman, R., Duttagupta, S., Mastey, V., Lloyd, J. R., & Fillit, H. (2002). Alzheimer's disease and related dementias increase costs of comorbidities in managed Medicare. *Neurology, 58,* 62–70.

Inouye, S. K., Bogardus, S. T., Vitagliano, G., Desai M. M., Williams, C. S., & Grady, et al. (2003). Burden of illness score for elderly persons: Risk adjustment incorporating the cumulative impact of diseases, physiologic abnormalities, and functional impairments. *Medical Care, 41*(1), 70–83.

Kales, H. C., Blow, F. C., Copeland, L. A., Bingham, R. C., Kammerer, E. E., & Mellow, A. M. (1999). Health care utilization by older patients with coexisting dementia and depression. *American Journal of Psychiatry, 156*(4), 550–556.

Kane, R. L., & Atherly, A. (2000). Medicare expenditures associated with Alzheimer's disease. *Alzheimer Disease and Associated Disorders, 14*(4), 187–195.

Kasper, J. D. (1995). Cognitive impairment in older people and use of physician services and inpatient care. In J. M. Wiener, S. B. Clauser, & D. L. Kennell (Eds.), *Persons with disabilities: Issues in health care financing and service delivery.* Washington, DC: Brookings Institution.

Kunik, M. E., Snow, A. L., Molinari, V. A., Menke, T. J., Souchek, J., & Sullivan G., et al. (2003). Health care utilization in dementia patients with psychiatric comorbidity. *Gerontologist, 43*(1), 86–91.

Leibson, C., Owens, T., O'Brien, P., Waring, S., Tangalos, E., & Hanson, V., et al. (1999). Use of physician and acute care services by persons with and without Alzheimer's disease: A population-based comparison. *Journal of the American Geriatrics Society, 47*(7), 864–869.

Lyketsos, C. G., Sheppard, J. E., & Rabins, P. V. (2000). Dementia in elderly persons in a general hospital. *American Journal of Psychiatry, 157*(5), 704–707.

Martin, B. C., Ricci, J. F., Kotzan, J. A., Lang, K., & Menzin, J. (2000). The net cost of Alzheimer disease and related dementia: A population-based study of Georgia Medicaid recipients. *Alzheimer Disease and Associated Disorders, 14*(3), 151–159.

Maslow, K. (2004). Dementia and serious coexisting medical conditions: A double whammy. *Nursing Clinics of North America, 39,* 561–579.

McCormick, W. C., Hardy, J., Kukull, W. A., Bowen, J. D., Teri, L., & Zitzer, S., et al. (2001). Healthcare utilization and costs in managed care patients with Alzheimer's disease during the last few years of life. *Journal of the American Geriatrics Society, 49*(9), 1156–1160.

McCormick, W. C., Kukull, W. A., Van Belle, G., Bowen, J. D., Teri, L., & Larson, E. B. (1995). The effect of diagnosing Alzheimer's disease on frequency of physician visits: A case-control study. *Journal of General Internal Medicine, 10,* 187–193.

Menzin, J., Lang, K., Friedman, M., Neumann, P., & Cummings, J. L. (1999). The economic cost of Alzheimer's disease and related dementias to the California Medicaid program ('Medi-Cal') in 1995. *American Journal of Geriatric Psychiatry, 7*(4), 300–308.

Murray, A. M., Levkoff, S. E., Wetle, T. T., Beckett, L., Cleary, P. D., & Schor, J. D., et al. (1993). Acute delirium and functional decline in the hospitalized elderly patient. *Journal of Gerontology: Medical Sciences, 48*(5), M181–M186.

Pompei, P., Foreman, M., Rudberg, M. A., Inouye, S. K., Braund, V., & Cassel, C. K. (1994). Delirium in hospitalized older persons: Outcomes and predictors. *Journal of the American Geriatrics Society, 42*(8), 809–815.

Rice, D. P., Fox, P. J., Max, W., Webber, P. A., Lindeman, D. A., & Hauck, W. W., et al. (1993). The economic burden of Alzheimer's disease. *Health Affairs, 12*(2), 164–176.

Richards, K. M., Shepherd, M. D., Crismon, M. L., Snyder, E. H., & Jermain, D. M. (2000). Medical services utilization and charge comparisons between elderly patients with and without Alzheimer's disease in a managed care organization. *Clinical Therapeutics, 22*(6), 775–206.

Sands, L. P., Yaffe, K., Covinsky, K., Chren, M-M., Counsell, S., & Palmer, R., et al. (2003). Cognitive screening predicts magnitude of functional recovery from admission to 3 months after discharge in hospitalized elders. *Journal of Gerontology: Medical Sciences, 58A*(1), 37–45.

Sloan, F. A., & Taylor, D. H. (2002). Effect of Alzheimer disease on the cost of treating other disease. *Alzheimer Disease and Associated Disorders, 16*(3), 137–143.

Taylor, D. H., & Sloan, F. A. (2000). How much do persons with Alzheimer's disease cost Medicare? *Journal of the American Geriatrics Society, 48*(6), 639–646.

Walsh, E. G., Wu, B., Mitchell, J. B., & Berkmann, L. F. (2003). Cognitive function and acute care utilization. *Journal of Gerontology: Social Sciences, 58B*(1), S38–S49.

Weiler, P. G., Lubben, J. E., & Chi, I. (1991). Cognitive impairment and hospital use. *American Journal of Public Health, 81*(9), 1153–1157.

Weiner, M., Powe, N. R., Weller, W. E., Shaffer, T. J., & Anderson, G. F. (1998). Alzheimer's disease under managed care: Implications from Medicare utilization and expenditure patterns. *Journal of the American Geriatrics Society, 46*(6), 762–770.

Welch, H. G., Walsh, J. S., & Larson, E. B. (1992). The cost of institutional care in Alzheimer's disease: Nursing home and hospital use in a prospective cohort. *Journal of the American Geriatrics Society, 40*(3), 21–224.

Wieland, D., Lamb, V. L., Sutton, S. R., Boland, R., Clark, M., & Friedman, S., et al. (2000). Hospitalization in the program of all-inclusive care for the elderly (PACE): Rates, concomitants, and predictors. *Journal of the American Geriatrics Society, 48*(11), 1373–1380.

CHAPTER TWO

In Search of Dementia-Friendly Hospitals

A Survey of Patient Care Directors in Massachusetts

Nina M. Silverstein

In 2000, about 9% of Medicare beneficiaries had at least one claim with a diagnostic code of Alzheimer's or dementia. These individuals had over three times more hospital stays than the average stays for all Medicare beneficiaries. Thus, these data suggest that there are over three million or more hospitalizations annually of persons with dementia (Alzheimer's Association, 2003).

Most hospitals probably are not prepared for this large number of elderly patients with dementia. Moreover, hospital administrators may not view their institutions as acute care settings for persons with dementia, but the Medicare data alert us to the fact that such patients are occupying their beds.

This chapter describes insights gained through a study conducted in 2000 at the University of Massachusetts Boston. The purpose of the research project was to gather data on current practices and planned changes regarding the care of patients with dementia, and to discern perceptions of patient care directors about the major challenges faced in providing such care. We sought answers to the questions, How "visible" were patients with dementia in Massachusetts' hospitals? and Was their dementia considered in their treatment plans for the duration of their hospital stays and in their discharge plans?

The study became an exploration of how *dementia-friendly* hospital stays are for persons with Alzheimer's disease or a related dementia. To operationalize dementia-friendly, we turned to the definition used by the national Alzheimer's Association.

The Alzheimer's Association (1997) has defined agencies that serve elders as dementia-specific, dementia-capable, or dementia-friendly. Dementia-specific agencies are those that serve individuals with Alzheimer's disease or a related disorder exclusively. Dementia-capable agencies are those that have staff trained in dementia care but also serve elders who are not cognitively impaired. Dementia-friendly agencies are agencies that serve all elders but do not have staff members specifically trained in dementia care. It seemed reasonable to consider this paradigm in thinking about hospitals—they do, after all, serve all elders and may not have staff members that are specifically trained in dementia care.

METHODOLOGY AND DATA COLLECTION

This research project was not externally funded; rather, it was conducted within the context of the requirements of gerontological undergraduate education at the University of Massachusetts Boston. In fall 1999 through spring 2000, the author led a two-semester seminar for undergraduate gerontology majors and advanced certificate students in gerontological social policy at the University of Massachusetts Boston, College of Public and Community Service (CPCS). The title of the seminar was "How Dementia-Friendly Are Acute Care Hospital Stays in Massachusetts?" The research design was conceptualized, and the specific domains to include in the questionnaire were defined during that first semester critical inquiry. During the second semester, ten students conducted the research project and interviewed directors of patient care (or their equivalents) in acute care hospitals in Massachusetts.[1] (For more information on CPCS and competency-based education, visit www.cpcs.umb.edu).

A semistructured interview schedule was designed to gather data on current practices and planned changes related to the care of patients with dementia in addition to gauging perceptions of the major chal-

---

[1]The following students are acknowledged for their contributions to this study: K. Goldberg, K. Greenan, P. Hogan, U. Kabba, M. Lojek, M. MacDonald, J. MacNeill, D. Pohotsky, J. Toomey, and J. Weistrop. Graduate assistant L. Bruner-Canhoto assisted with data analysis.

lenges faced in providing care to patients with dementia. The ten students were charged with identifying a convenience sample of hospitals to visit across Massachusetts. A letter describing the study and seeking cooperation preceded the in-person interview. The response to participate in the study was very favorable, with most respondents recognizing the issue and wanting to share their experiences.

RESULTS FROM THE PILOT STUDY[2]

Sample Description

In-person interviews were conducted with thirty-three directors of patient care during spring 2000. Thirty-two of the thirty-three hospitals were in Massachusetts. The final hospital was on the border of Massachusetts and New Hampshire and, technically, in New Hampshire. Forty-two percent (fourteen hospitals) were affiliated with another medical facility or health provider group. Thirty percent (ten hospitals) had affiliations with nursing homes ranging from associations with two to thirty nursing homes. Four of the hospitals were private nonprofit orthopedic facilities. The hospitals ranged in size from 50 acute care beds to over 600 beds. The staff-to-patient ratio varied from 1:4 to 1:7 during the day and slightly lower at night. The approximate number of in-patient admissions per month ranged from 36 to 2,000 patients and averaged between 300 and 500 patients.

Dementia Patient Caseload

To address the question of how visible patients with dementia were in acute hospital settings, we wanted to know if they were "counted"; that is, was their dementia status noted in their admission records?

When asked how many patients with dementia were in the current patient caseload, most hospital personnel could not state how many were currently admitted in their hospitals. It appeared that dementia was not consistently recorded on patients' records. However, when asked to give their best estimate of patients with dementia who are currently hospitalized, most were at least able to offer estimated percentages. Those estimates, however, were not terribly useful because the estimated percentages reported of patients with dementing illnesses who were admitted each month ranged broadly from 5 to 75%. For many, it was the first time they were asked to consider the number of patients with dementia.

---

[2]These data were originally presented in poster format at the Alzheimer's Association, Massachusetts Chapter Professional Education Conference, May 2000.

Now that the interviewees were focused on dementia, they were able to respond to the question of the relative change observed in the patient case-load and offered responses to the question, Within the past five years, would you say there has been an increase, a decrease, or has the number of patients with dementia remained the same? As Figure 2.1 shows, 45% of those interviewed said that they had observed an increase in the number of patients with dementia in the past five years; 40% felt that the census had not changed; 3% thought it had decreased; and 12% reported that they did not know.

Only one of the respondents indicated that a mental status assessment was conducted as a routine part of the intake exam for adult patients at the time of admissions. Three others said that a mental status assessment is conducted on an "as needed" basis. The specific content of the mental status assessment was not described.

Five of the hospitals noted that they had specific admissions policies for patients when the hospital was aware of the existence of dementing illnesses. The following is an example of how a policy was described:

> *A day or two before admission, if possible, we take the patient's history, conduct a physical and mental assessment, and various testing.*

A detailed and "specific" protocol per se did not truly exist.

We then asked whether the hospitals had specific admission policies for patients who manifest extreme behavioral changes. The responses were quite varied:

> *Not specific—falls within regular policy.*
> *Sent for psych evaluation.*
> *Seek immediate involvement with social services.*
> *Placed in observation rooms near nursing stations.*
> *Move patient to private room.*
> *A nurse is assigned or a family caregiver must stay with the patient.*
> *Transfer patient to another setting.*

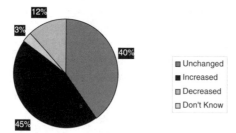

FIGURE 2.1 Change in prevalence of dementia patients (n = 33). Hospital personnel were asked to give an opinion on whether the percentage of patients with dementing illnesses has changed.

Staff Training

We were interested in learning whether the staff received specialized training in dementia care and which staff members were likely to receive such training. Were they prepared to meet the needs of a patient who might wander away from a reception area, emergency room, or hospital bed? Did they know about community-based programs and services that train staff members in dementia care in order to make appropriate referrals upon discharge?

The format of the staff training that was reported was typically training conducted as part of a one-time in-service workshop or covered within an orientation program for newly hired staff. Intensive training in dementia care was not mentioned by any of the hospitals. Moreover, five of the hospitals reported that no specific training was offered in dementia care. Of those staff members who were trained, nurses and social workers were most likely to receive any type of specialized training (88%), followed by nurse's aides (85%) and physicians (61%). The specific content or duration of the training sessions was not described. Thus, for our analysis purposes, attending a multisession course or a noontime lecture was counted as receiving "specialized training."

It is interesting that volunteers, custodial, and security personnel, all groups likely to come in direct contact with patients, were least likely to receive any type of specialized training (3%). Training such persons is especially important in managing behaviors such as wandering, falls, and agitation.

All interviewers reported enthusiasm among those interviewed for more information on the topic of caring for the patient with dementia in an acute care setting. Specifically, there was great interest among those interviewed for more training in dementia care. The interviewees identified several topics in which they would like to receive more training:

- Meal-time concerns related to proper techniques for assistance with feeding; increased knowledge on nutritional needs as well as understanding "dementia-friendly" food
- Maintenance of prehospital continence and mobility
- Fall prevention
- Limiting restraint use
- Legal issues including the process for assigning guardianship through the courts
- End-of-life care
- Discharge planning

The gerontology students observed that throughout the interview, the respondents appeared to sincerely appreciate the opportunity to reflect on concerns they had regarding the care of patients with dementia. They identified major challenges they encounter in providing quality care, best summarized as *communication, managing difficult behaviors*, and *safety*.

Communication was noted as a challenge not only in reference to communicating with the patient but also in talking to family members. As anyone who has visited a hospital knows, there is a great deal of paperwork to complete in the process of seeking care. This necessary task is difficult to perform without the assistance of a family member or other patient advocate. It was noted that it was difficult for patients to complete financial forms and to apply for financial aid without family assistance in the application process.

A specific concern voiced with regard to decision-making was the question of who should be contacted. Most patients are admitted without family members or contact persons noted in their records. The lack of a primary contact was especially disconcerting when questions about end-of-life care decisions arose. The interviewees expressed difficulty understanding patient needs; monitoring their pain; and dealing with issues when there was a lack of consent or health care proxy.

Managing difficult behaviors was also a great frustration for the interviewees. They expressed that patients with dementia were physically demanding, needing hands-on care for basic needs and all activities of daily living (ADLs). They asked for guidance on keeping patients calm and managing agitation and confusion.

Safety was mentioned as a major challenge. Specifically, the interviewees were concerned about keeping patients safe without using restraints. Many of those interviewed asked for a copy of the questionnaire used in the interview since several questions related to creating a supportive environment, and this topic generated a good deal of discussion that the interviewees wanted to share with other staff members. They were specifically interested in modifications that could be made to the environment such as lighting, positioning of the bed, noise control, and exit control.

The concern for safety was also raised in regard to finding appropriate placements for discharge. Locating a bed at an appropriate rehab or nursing home at time of discharge was a challenge noted by several of the interviewees.

Knowledge of Safe Return™

Safe Return™ is a wanderers' alert program sponsored by the Alzheimer's Association in cooperation with the U.S. Justice Department. The program was legislated by Congress in 1992 in an effort to address the individual protection problems associated with wandering behavior in Alzheimer's disease. It is a proactive program designed to safely return missing persons with Alzheimer's disease and related disorders and to train police, emergency personnel, and others to recognize the dangers associated with wandering behavior and to deal appropriately with them (Silverstein, Flaherty, & Tobin, 2002).

The majority of the respondents (85%) in our pilot study were either not aware of or unsure if they knew about the Safe Return™ program (Figure 2.2). Moreover, none of the hospitals reported having a specific policy or lost person's protocol in place to refer to when a patient wandered away. Safe Return™ recommends searching the premises for 15 minutes from the point of last seen (PLS) and then calling the police and then notifying Safe Return™. Planning the procedure that hospital staff might follow in those 15 minutes is critical to maximizing the possibility of a rapid and safe recovery of a missing patient with dementia. Examples of steps to include in a lost person's protocol can be adapted from those described for long-term care settings in Silverstein, Flaherty, and Tobin (2002).

Some patients with dementia arrive at the hospital emergency department when they are found wandering by law enforcement personnel, lacking identification for returning them home. We asked, What is the procedure for assessment and disposition when a patient with a dementing illness is found wandering in the community and is brought to the emergency department by law enforcement personnel? Clear and specific protocols were lacking across all of the respondents' hospitals. Three interviewees mentioned that they would contact the Alzheimer's Association. Others noted working with the police to ID the patient and locate family members; and still others responded that they evaluate and keep the patient safe while law enforcement tries to locate the family. A few mentioned involving their social services departments early on or seeking psychiatric evaluation. Almost all of the respondents had experience with this situation—only three indicated that they had not. Checking for

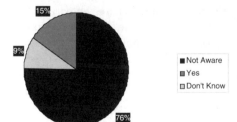

FIGURE 2.2   Knowledge of Safe Return™ (n = 33). Hospital personnel were asked if they were aware of the Safe Return™ program, a wanderers' alert program sponsored by the National Alzheimer's Association.

Safe Return™ identification (a bracelet or necklace) and contacting the trained professionals associated with the program would be helpful steps to list in a hospital's protocol for procedures to take when a patient with dementia elopes. Three of the respondents specifically asked to have information about the Safe Return™ program sent to them.

To assure continuity of care from the hospital to community, we included questions related to discharge planning. Specifically, we asked if staff were knowledgeable of services in the community for persons with dementia. Just over a third (twelve hospitals) responded affirmatively. For these hospitals, the staff members most knowledgeable of community-based care were the social workers, case managers, and chaplains. Four of the hospitals reported that they involve community providers in designing their discharge plans.

The interviewer continued by asking if the hospitals had programs or referred patients to programs that slowly introduce restorative function. Forty-two percent (fourteen hospitals) said that they either have their own inpatient rehabilitation units or that they refer, although it was not clear from the interviews how much the rehabilitation units were used for patients with dementia. Three more hospitals indicated that it was a future goal, in the talking stages, or that newer policies are about to be introduced.

Adaptations to Care Practice and to the Environment

None of the hospitals had special care units or ACE (acute care for the elderly) sections where they were likely to place patients with dementing illnesses who had acute care needs, although one hospital did have plans to develop such a unit. The general response was that patients are admitted to the unit that best addresses their medical needs. One respondent reported that her hospital had a purple sticker program for fall risk. Several respondents in our pilot study noted adaptations they had made in care practices or in the environment. It was striking that whether or not the dementia itself was defined from the outset, once the patient reached the unit, the nursing staff did make some adaptations that acknowledged the dementia. Almost all, 97%, reported that they select a room in a quieter area of the nursing unit where the patient has to pass by the nursing station before reaching an exit. Eighty percent encouraged the selection of a private room to control noise and extraneous stimuli. Over half (58%) positioned the bed to minimize visible cues of exits. Other adaptations noted by interviewees in this study were the use of alarms or buzzers, regular patient checks or "sweeps," alarm strips placed on bed and chairs, and wanderers' gowns (separate color than usual hospital gowns). Two respondents reported having safe rooms with special beds and wander alarms. Still other adaptations related to responding to challenging behaviors by playing music, having a game box, or encouraging the patient to sit in a rocking chair. Most of the interviewees reported a minimal use of restraints or using them as a last resort. Several mentioned that they start with the least restrictive device.

In general, the hospitals were very interested in learning about environmental modifications and changes in care practice that might be useful in caring for patients with dementia. Many asked for copies of the survey items related to the environment and asked to have additional materials on environmental adaptations mailed to them following the interview.

Family Involvement

All of the interviewees said that they include family members at some level in the care plan development. Some reported in-person contact while others said that they speak to family members by telephone. One hospital offered daily conferences with the care team. Another respondent said that they do not involve family unless a problem exists. Still others reported that they involve families only to plan discharge arrangements. Almost all, 91%, reported that they allow family members to stay with the patient overnight. One hospital noted that they supply meals and a bed for family members. Two-thirds noted that they routinely conduct family meetings with health care providers regarding patients with dementing illnesses. Specific challenges noted included the need to improve their ability to locate family members, to educate family members regarding dementia, and to educate family members on the importance of seeking legal advice on issues such as end-of-life care and durable power of attorney for medical decisions. Families were also encouraged to hire private duty nurses or sitters to stay overnight with patients.

Supervision is a critical component in dementia care. In a busy hospital setting, 24-hour supervision or surveillance might not always be possible. The interviewees were asked if their hospitals have sitter services and if those services were provided by volunteer or paid staff. Most of the hospitals had staff available for hire; some of the hospitals provided aides, while one of the larger hospitals was in the process of setting up a separate sitter service.

When asked if the hospitals kept a pool of private duty nurses to recommend to families, only one hospital responded affirmatively that such a list is kept but that the families must make their own arrangements. Other hospitals noted that they recommend agencies but do not provide individual names.

Utilization of Volunteers

The majority, 79%, reported that they used volunteers to assist with patients. For the most part, volunteers assisted by transporting patients within the hospital (88%). Over half, 54%, of those who used volunteers, did so to provide supervision and companionship. One of the hospitals had a volunteer storyteller who visited and entertained the patients. Just over one-third, 35%, used volunteers to assist with feeding. This latter point generated much discussion related to the liability associated with patients who might aspirate. To address this concern, one of the larger hospitals was planning a seminar to train volunteers to assist with feeding. In contrast, one hospital reported that the volunteers do not have any direct contact with patients—they are only used in the gift shop or the library.

Participation in Research

The respondents were asked if their hospital participated in formal research regarding dementing illnesses (Figure 2.3). Three of the hospitals were currently involved with research projects while one was in the planning stages. Of those hospitals, one had a division of gerontology and offered an internship program for nurses who were specializing in the care of patients with dementia; a second hospital had a neurology department that had on-going research in dementia; and the third hospital reported having two doctors actively involved in research on aging, with one current project specifically examining caregiving relationships among older women. Another question related to research was whether the hospitals made information available to caregivers about brain autopsy. Six of the respondents reported that they do make that information available indirectly through the organ bank and not directly through the hospital.

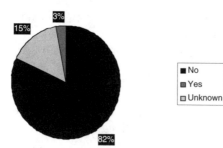

FIGURE 2.3   Participation in formal research. Hospital personnel were asked if their facility participated in formal research regarding dementing illnesses.

CONCLUSION

The pilot study served to raise awareness of the issue of persons with dementia who are hospitalized for their acute care needs. It was a learning experience not only for the student interviewers but also for the hospital personnel who gave their time to participate in the study. Many asked for a copy of the questionnaire, particularly for the information regarding environmental features. All identified with the issue and acknowledged great challenges and the need for new strategies to address those challenges. All seemed interested in expanded training opportunities to increase their knowledge and expertise in caring for the acute care needs of patients with dementia. The major recommendation to emerge from these data is the need for hospitals to develop or adapt protocols that recognize and consider the specialized needs of the patient with dementia in the areas of admission, in-patient care, and discharge planning, in addition to being prepared for episodes of elopement by following lost person protocols that are consistent with the procedures recommended by Safe Return™.

REFERENCES

Alzheimer's Association. (1997). *Community assessment workbook for dementia services*. Chicago, IL: Alzheimer's Association.

Alzheimer's Association. (2003). *Use of Medicare services and Medicare costs for people with Alzheimer's disease and dementia—2000*. Washington, DC: Alzheimer's Association.

Silverstein, N. M., Flaherty, G., & Tobin, T. S. (2002). *Dementia and wandering behavior: Concern for the lost elder*. New York: Springer, 215 pp.

CHAPTER THREE

Acute Care for Nursing Home Residents with Alzheimer's Disease

Understanding Variations in Hospital Use Rates

Mary W. Carter and Frank W. Porell

THE NURSING HOME SETTING

Although frequently considered the "last stop" along the health care continuum, nursing homes form a crucial link in the overall structure and delivery of health care services for frail elders, including management of chronic and disabling conditions; provision of long-term social and medical supports; assistance with activities of daily living; coordination of rehabilitative services aimed at restoring independent functioning; and provision of palliative care at the end-of-life. Thus, nursing homes typically serve diverse populations with equally varied health care needs, necessitating the provision of a broad spectrum of services on a daily basis and within a single setting.

Currently, approximately 17,000 nursing homes are in operation across the United States, serving an estimated 1.56 million residents aged 65 years and older. Most nursing homes are Medicare and/or Medicaid certified (95%), operate as for-profit ventures (67%), and are chain-affiliated (56%) (Gabrel, 2000a). The typical long-stay resident has resided in the same nursing home for a little more than two years (Dey, 1997), is approximately 84 years of age, female (75%), widowed (63%) (Gabrel, 2000b), and requires nursing assistance for multiple comorbidities and assistance with three or more activities of daily living, such as eating, bathing, transferring, toileting, and dressing (Gabrel, 2000b). Additionally, approximately half of all nursing home residents have Alzheimer's disease or a related dementia (ADRD) (Rhoades, Potter, & Krauss, 1998).

Despite the comprehensive array of services provided by nursing homes, nursing homes are not isolated operations, but instead interact continuously with other health care providers such as short-stay hospitals, rehabilitation facilities, assisted living units, and home health care agencies, to name a few. Along this continuum of care, frequent transfers occur between health care settings, especially between nursing homes and short-stay hospitals (Freiman & Murtaugh, 1995). The growing frequency of this specific relationship reflects changing policies over the past 30 years, including implementation of Medicare and Medicaid, the Prospective Payment System, and the Omnibus Budget Reconciliation Act of 1987 (Liu, Wissoker, & Rimes, 1998; Rubenstein, Ouslander, & Wieland, 1988). Following changes in hospital reimbursement policies stemming from the implementation of the Prospective Payment System (PPS) in 1983, levels of illness severity and complexity of care needs have steadily increased among nursing home residents. In part, these changes are thought to be attributable to shorter hospital stays resulting in patients being discharged earlier in the recovery process with subsequently greater levels of patient acuity. Greater acuity levels at the time of hospital discharge have lead to increased reliance upon post-acute, long-term care, which in turn has demanded that the long-term care industry supply progressively more complex and technically sophisticated care to an often older and more medically needy population (Bergman & Clarfield, 1991; Buchanan, Madel, & Persons, 1991; Holtzman & Lurie et al., 1996; Liu, Wissoker, & Rimes, 1998). Consequently, although the nursing home has always formed a crucial link in the overall structure and delivery of health care services to frail elders, common care practices now include intermittent transfers from the nursing home to the hospital for episodes of acute care to meet the increasing health care demands of the nursing home population.

THE NURSING HOME/HOSPITAL CONNECTION

Over the past two decades clinicians, researchers, and policymakers have increasingly expressed concern regarding the frequency with which residents of nursing homes are transferred to hospitals for acute care. Although reported hospitalization rates vary as much as fivefold across the extant literature (Castle & Mor, 1996), recent estimates from the 1997 National Nursing Home Survey indicate that approximately 28% of all nursing home residents are discharged annually at least once to a short-term acute care hospital (Gabrel, 2000b), with a subset of residents experiencing multiple hospitalizations over a relatively short period of time (Coburn, Keith, & Bolda, 2002).

In addition to the exorbitant health care costs associated with hospitalizations, short-term transfers from the nursing home to the hospital also may involve considerable disruption and relocation stress (Ouslander, 1988), complicate existing and/or trigger new illnesses (Spector & Takada, 1991), result in new or worsening pressure sores (Berlowitz, Brandeis, Anderson, & Brand, 1997), and may be followed by irreversible, functional decline (Creditor, 1993). Given the seriousness of each of these possibilities, recent efforts to understand factors associated with hospitalization rates and sources of variation in hospital use rates across nursing homes have been undertaken, with a particular interest in identifying potential areas for reducing unnecessary and/or potentially avoidable hospitalizations among nursing home residents. Although these studies have imparted valuable insight regarding resident- and facility-level determinants of hospitalization, to date only a few studies have explored how these factors affect hospitalization risk among specific subpopulations of the nursing home, such as residents with ADRD, and fewer still have considered potentially avoidable and/or discretionary hospitalizations of nursing home residents with ADRD.

HOSPITALIZATION RATES AMONG RESIDENTS WITH ALZHEIMER'S DISEASE: A PARADOX?

Residents with ADRD represent a particularly vulnerable nursing home subpopulation. For example, residents with ADRD experience increased risk of malnutrition, dehydration (Burger, Kayser-Jones, & Bell, 2000), and injurious falls/fractures (Rubenstein, Josephson, & Osterweil, 1996), are more likely to be physically restrained (Sullivan-Mark, Strumpf, Evans, Baumgarten & Maislin, 1999), and are less likely to receive analgesics to relieve pain symptoms (Won, Lapane, Gambassi, Bernabei, Mor, & Lipsitz, 1999). Such outcomes have been shown to increase a nursing home resident's risk of being hospitalized (e.g., Carter & Porell, 2003; Zimmerman, Gruber-Baldini, Hebel, Sloane, & Magaziner, 2002), as well as the length of the hospital stay once admitted (Burger, Kayser-Jones, & Bell, 2000). However, despite the higher incidence of these hospitalization risk factors among nursing home residents with ADRD, current research suggests that residents with ADRD experience no greater, and perhaps even a lower, hospitalization risk than do residents without ADRD (Fried & Mor, 1997; Murtaugh & Freiman, 1995).

The apparent lower hospitalization risk of ADRD residents suggests an interesting paradox in light of some recent study findings. For example, Burton and colleagues (2001) followed residents quarterly for approximately three years after nursing home admission and found that residents with ADRD consistently received fewer physician visits in comparison with residents without ADRD. The authors also report that residents with ADRD are less likely to be seen by a physician or hospitalized for the treatment of an infection compared with residents without ADRD. Further research findings suggest that although residents with ADRD do not appear any more likely to be hospitalized in general, when residents with ADRD are hospitalized, the admitting diagnosis is more likely to be classified as ambulatory care sensitive, suggesting that problems may potentially exist for nursing home residents with ADRD in terms of access to adequate and timely health care services necessary for the optimal treatment of their chronic conditions (Carter, 2003a).

THE POLICY CONUNDRUM

Despite the apparent tendency for nursing home residents with ADRD to be hospitalized less frequently than residents without ADRD, the causes and consequences of this pattern are not well understood. Some researchers have suggested that the less frequent rates of hospitalization among residents with AD may reflect end-of-life decisions to seek less aggressive and more palliative health care options (e.g., Fillenbaum, Heyman, Peterson, Pieper, & Weiman, 2001); other researchers have focused more specifically on various health outcomes, such as weight loss, rates of infection, and decline in physical functioning, and have concluded that more intensive preventative care approaches are needed (Sloss, Solomon, Shekelle, Young, Salibar, & MacLean, et al., 2000).

Moreover, although preventing potentially avoidable and unnecessary hospitalizations among nursing home residents represents an important health policy goal, most studies investigating hospitalization patterns among nursing home residents have tended to focus only on the suspected problem of overutilization of acute care services among nursing home residents, and in turn, have recommended reducing overall rates of hospitalization rather than targeting specific types of preventable or unnecessary hospitalizations. Overutilization of acute care services may expose nursing home residents to unnecessary relocation stress, iatrogenic illnesses, and irreversible decline, as well as result in wasted resources and exorbitant expenses. Less frequently considered, however, are those effects stemming from under-utilization of acute care services, which may include needless pain and suffering, unnecessary medical complications, and physical or mental deterioration, as well as inefficient use of limited nursing home resources. Accordingly, public policies designed solely to reduce overall hospitalization rates among nursing home residents risk implementing containment strategies that potentially could limit medically necessary hospitalizations at the same rate as medically unnecessary hospitalizations. Such an approach would most likely have particularly serious consequences for nursing home residents with ADRD who, because of the clinical nature of their disease, such as memory impairments, cognitive deficits, and mood/behavior changes, are dependent on the nursing home for the management and provision of day-to-day medical and direct physical care.

Moreover, research suggests that the facility in which a resident lives and the market characteristics of the area where the nursing home is located may be as important as the particular care needs of a given resident in determining whether or not a hospitalization occurs. In other words, population differences in health care needs across nursing homes fail to explain differences in hospitalization rates among nursing home residents. Most likely, this is because factors other than resident illness levels, such as facility structural attributes or area-market factors, contribute to the differential hospitalization rates as well.

Additionally, the actual decision regarding whether or not a nursing home resident is hospitalized most likely rests with two parties. First, a member of the nursing home staff must bring to a physician's attention (either via telephone or transport) the resident's medical need. Second, once notified, the physician must then decide whether in-hospital treatment versus nursing home–based treatment is warranted. Because of the fragmentation of services across providers and the different sources of reimbursement and regulation governing both providers, decisions to hospitalize reflect a complex set of system incentives, of which clinical need may be only one aspect. The extent to which variations in hospitalization rates stem from provider differences in decision-making may be further confounded by the degree to which nursing home facilities lack needed equipment and have sufficient numbers of adequately trained personnel to care for individual health care needs.

Nursing home residents with ADRD are particularly vulnerable to such variations because of their reliance on skilled nursing care and daily provision of supportive therapies to avoid further worsening of symptoms. Thus, when the system relied upon to provide medical assistance for optimal functioning actually contributes to the risk of unnecessary or preventable hospitalizations, identification of these risk factors is critical to improving hospitalization practices in the nursing home to achieve improved resident outcomes.

HOSPITALIZATION PATTERNS OF NURSING HOME RESIDENTS: WHAT WE KNOW

Although at times hospitalization clearly may be in a nursing home resident's best interest, especially when preferred treatment options are not available in the nursing home, researchers and medical professionals have more frequently argued that the frequency of hospitalization is too high (Fried & Mor, 1997). In response to this concern, most studies have focused on individual-level predictors of hospital use, while tending to define hospitalization in terms of a simple dichotomy, that is, whether or not a hospitalization occurred. Consequently, few studies have examined facility- or market-area determinants of resident transfers to hospitals, and fewer still have explored whether differential effects exist for vulnerable subpopulations in the nursing home, such as residents with ADRD. Thus, although a body of empirical research exploring factors associated with increased hospitalization risk among nursing home residents has begun to be assembled, more attention is needed to explicate the complicated relationship between various sets of factors and their relationships to hospitalization, particularly for vulnerable populations. Nonetheless, despite the fact that most of the research has not focused specifically on Alzheimer's disease, the findings discussed in this section provide some notable insights relevant to residents with ADRD in terms of the types of factors that, in general, contribute to hospital admission among nursing home residents.

Early studies of causes of hospitalization among nursing home residents tended to rely on small study samples and medical chart review methodologies to determine whether nursing home residents were being unnecessarily transferred to hospitals, and whether adverse consequences were observed upon their return. Overall, findings suggest that genitourinary infections, respiratory disorders, cerebral vascular diseases, gastrointestinal disorders, congestive heart failure, fractures, and infections are the leading medical conditions requiring hospitalization among nursing home residents. While this profile of medical conditions generally reflects the hospitalization experience of ADRD residents, these residents appear to be hospitalized more frequently for potentially avoidable infectious conditions such as bacterial pneumonia, gastroenteritis, and kidney and urinary tract infections, particularly in nursing homes with high overall hospitalization rates among all residents (Carter & Porell, 2003b).

Findings also suggest that, upon return to the nursing home, residents are more likely to have developed a pressure ulcer during their hospitalization compared with residents without a hospitalization, and many of those hospitalized will experience a repeat hospitalization within the following thirty days. This has important implications for residents with ADRD since they are at greater risk of developing pressure ulcers than other nursing home residents (Volicer & Hurley 1997). Finally, a few studies have suggested that lack of onsite medical services, such as radiology and laboratory equipment, add to the risk of hospitalization and that the availability of such services combined with facility resources to monitor and administer intravenous fluids could prevent many hospitalizations from occurring (e.g., Kayser-Jones, Wiener, & Barbaccia, 1989).

A later study, performed by Teresi and colleagues (1991), attempted to identify facility-level attributes associated with high versus low hospital transfer rates. While the authors concluded that certain structural attributes, such as 24-hour nurse staffing and the availability of in-house intravenous therapy, probably prevented some transfers, they note the critical role of physicians in determining hospital transfer. The authors suggested that variations in hospital transfer rates arise in larger part from considerable differences in physicians' tolerance for managing medically complex procedures in the nursing home versus the hospital, fear of malpractice complaints, and responsiveness to broader system incentives such as higher reimbursement rates. To the extent that ADRD residents are less able to effectively communicate their needs and medical preferences, this interpretation of their findings suggests that physician preferences are likely to have even greater influence on transfer decisions for ADRD residents than for other residents.

Although case studies can provide a valuable glimpse into the causes of hospitalization at a given point in time, studies drawing upon large, secondary data sources allow for analysis of the effects of structural and contextual factors stemming from the organizational arrangement of care (e.g., proprietary status), and perhaps the interaction of these factors with individual resident characteristics, on resident hospitalization risk. The cumulative impacts of nonclinical structural and contextual factors on risk of hospitalization are quite large. After adjusting for resident case-mix differences, Carter and Porell (2003) found that a resident's risk of hospitalization varied by more than twofold among individual nursing homes in Massachusetts depending on characteristics of the facility and its location. Furthermore, even greater interfacility variations in hospitalization risk were found for ADRD residents than for residents without ADRD (Porell & Carter, 2003).

Although only a handful of studies have studied the influence of contextual factors, a rough picture of how contextual factors affect nursing home hospitalization rates has begun to emerge. For example, Freiman and Murtaugh (1993) report that nonprofit homes appear less likely to transfer residents to hospitals relative to for-profit homes, and increased reimbursement levels to nursing homes also appear to decrease resident risk of hospitalization. Mor and colleagues (1997) note that the introduction of the Resident Assessment Instrument (RAI)—a mandatory resident case management and documentation procedure in the nursing home, resulted in a 25% reduction in hospitalization rates between the years 1991 to 1993. This finding may suggest an interaction between resident-level medical needs and the organizational and structural response of the facility in meeting those needs. Intrator and colleagues (1999) reported that increased nursing home use of medical professionals, including physicians, nurse practitioners, and physician assistants, lowered hospitalization rates among nursing home residents. Recent findings from Carter (2003a) also highlight the important role of nurse staffing patterns with respect to hospitalization risk. Increased RN staffing levels were shown not only to decrease hospitalizations in general, but ambulatory care-sensitive hospitalizations in particular. This is important because the latter subgroup of hospitalizations stems from medical conditions thought to be largely preventable (e.g., diabetes, asthma, congestive heart failure) through timely access to outpatient physician and other medical support services.

Although few studies have attempted to link quality-of-care processes in the nursing home with resident risk of hospitalization, more than likely, differences in the delivery of care across nursing homes account for some of the observed variation in hospitalization rates. Fried and Mor (1997) identified several variables suggestive of nursing home care practices, such as percent of residents receiving new medications, with feeding tubes present, and with pressure ulcers (stage 2+), to be associated with increased risk of hospitalization. Carter and Porell (2002) estimate that the cumulative impact of nursing home performance on three quality-of-care indicators (presence of stage 2 and higher decubiti, physical restraint application, and unintentional weight loss) may account for as much as 43% of the observed difference in risk of hospitalization across nursing homes. Finally, other studies have linked nursing home performance on quality indicators to resident outcomes associated with increased hospitalization risk. Castle and Fogel (1998) found that nursing homes with higher levels of RN staffing and lower levels of LPN staffing were significantly less likely to use physical restraints. Considered together, these related study findings most likely bear particular significance for residents with ADRD, who are more likely to be physically restrained while in the nursing homes and who, potentially, may be monitored less intensely by licensed medical personnel in the nursing home for certain medical conditions (e.g., pneumonia) when compared with residents without ADRD.

UNDERSTANDING SOURCES OF VARIATION AND THEIR IMPLICATIONS FOR RESIDENTS WITH ALZHEIMER'S DISEASE AND RELATED DEMENTIAS

It seems clear that illness alone cannot account for the variation between nursing home transfer rates of residents to acute care hospitals. Instead, the effects of sociodemographic characteristics, such as age or gender, functional status factors, such as incontinence or cognitive impairment, and chronic diseases such as diabetes or Alzheimer's disease on hospitalization may be mitigated or accentuated, depending on the individual nursing home's structural and contextual characteristics. Onsite capacity for administration and monitoring of intravenous fluids in a nursing home can directly prevent some hospital transfers that would have occurred otherwise. Contextual factors may also indirectly influence hospitalization risk. A higher staffing level in a nursing home may better help residents to maintain independent ambulation by affording them more opportunities to ambulate (with or without assistance) and by lesser use of restraints in situations where assistance from multiple persons is warranted. Ambulation is particularly important for residents with ADRD in helping to prevent medical complications, such as urinary tract infections, pneumonia, and pressure ulcers that can result in hospitalization (Volicer, 2001). Thus, what may necessitate medical transfer in one facility may not in another facility, raising the important question: To what extent do variations in hospitalization rates reflect actual population differences across nursing homes versus differences in structural and organizational attributes across nursing homes, or even broader area market effects?

Despite the identification of important determinants of hospitalization, large unexplained variations in hospitalization practices across nursing homes persist. In response, new research efforts are investigating the extent to which practice style effects may contribute to the observed variations. Researchers interested in variations in hospital use among community-based populations have long suspected that, in part, hospital use variations reflect differences in practice styles among physicians (Wennberg, Barnes, & Zubkoff, 1982). Earlier studies have demonstrated that the extent to which practice style differences are observed through variations in hospitalization rates varies with the level of professional discretion associated with a particular condition (Roos, Wennberg, & McPherson, 1988). Here, the term "discretion" refers to the degree to which doctors face uncertainty regarding the use of in-hospital treatment versus other treatment options. For example, previous research has noted that certain medical conditions, such as acute myocardial infarction, have well-documented clinical guidelines and treatment protocols, resulting in relatively uniform treatment plans among physicians. Other conditions, however, such as chronic emphysema, lack widely established treatment standards and consequently entail greater levels of individual physician discretion in deciding whether or not to hospitalize (Roos et al., 1988). The more physicians disagree about appropriate treatment for a medical condition, the more likely local physician practice styles and supply factors, such as the availability of hospital beds, determine local rates of hospital use.

Physicians are likely to face greater uncertainties about the relative effectiveness of alternative diagnostic and therapeutic approaches for treating the acute illnesses of nursing home residents because of clinical differences from the larger community population. Dementia is likely to introduce additional complexities. Clinical information, such as medical histories, may be less reliable for some ADRD residents (Ouslander, 1989). Because of the recurrent nature of infections among individuals with ADRD, antibiotic therapy has limited effectiveness in treating pneumonia in this patient population (Fabiszewski, Volicer, & Volicer, 1990). Certain aggressive medical treatments, such as intravenous therapy, often require the use of physical or chemical restraints when administered to ADRD residents, which further increases their already high risk of developing pressure ulcers and contractures (Volicer, 2001). Dementia may also prevent patients from reporting severe discomfort or adverse effects of prescribed medications, essentially rendering them unable to participate in decisions regarding their own medical care (Ouslander, 1989). Accordingly, discretionary hospitalization practices in nursing homes appear to hold particularly important implications for nursing home residents with ADRD.

In a recent study investigating discretionary hospitalization practices for residents in nursing homes, the findings of Carter (2003b) indicated that when compared with otherwise similar residents, residents with Alzheimer's disease were more likely to be hospitalized for high discretion conditions. The researchers also examined the composition of hospitalizations occurring across nursing homes with overall high and low hospital transfer rates. Findings from these comparisons indicated that the proportion of high discretionary hospitalizations tended to increase as the overall number of hospitalizations increased across nursing homes, even though the proportion of low discretion hospitalizations remained relatively stable. In other words, it appears that nursing homes with higher hospitalization rates are hospitalizing residents more frequently for conditions recognized as involving a greater level of professional discretion in the decision to hospitalize. Finally, the study findings also impart some important insights about the medical conditions of nursing home residents with hospitalizations considered to be discretionary. The most frequent high discretion conditions cited in the study included congestive heart failure (23%), dehydration (13%), chronic obstructive pulmonary disease (6%), atrial fibrillation (3%), and cardiac dysrhythmias (2%) (Carter, 2003b). While there is a similar very high prevalence of hospitalizations for congestive heart failure among the community elderly, this prevalence of hospitalizations for dehydration among nursing home residents is notably high.

More recently, Porell and Carter (2005) undertook an in-depth examination of high discretion hospitalization practices for nursing home residents with ADRD. The study examined whether structural and organizational characteristics of nursing homes differentially affect high discretion hospitalization rates for residents with ADRD compared with residents from the same facility without ADRD. Several outcomes unique to residents with ADRD were found, including issues related to RN staffing levels, facility proprietary status and resident behavior and illness levels. For example, nursing home residents with ADRD of facilities that rely more heavily on temporary RN staffing from off-site agencies experienced greater odds of being transferred to a hospital for a high discretion condition than did residents who resided in facilities employing a more permanent base of RN staffing hours. Moreover, it appeared that increased staffing intensity of RNs helps to decrease high discretionary hospitalizations by reducing the number of hospitalizations that occur among the more severely ill residents with ADRD. Considering that similar results were not found for residents without ADRD, these findings, taken together, most likely indicate that familiarity among RN staff with a resident's history is particularly important for residents with Alzheimer's disease in preventing high discretionary hospitalizations, probably because of the difficulties in communicating with persons with ADRD. Reductions may occur because RNs who are familiar with residents may be better able to discern medical needs because of familiarity with the medical history, and may also be more supportive of palliative care efforts for those residents with complex medical nursing needs, resulting in fewer hospitalizations.

Further, findings from Porell and Carter (2005) also indicate that high discretion hospitalizations were more likely among residents with ADRD residing in for-profit nursing homes who either experienced an accident or who exhibited behavioral problems in comparison with otherwise similar residents located in nonprofit nursing homes. Likewise, ADRD residents with decubiti were also more likely to be hospitalized than were ADRD residents without decubiti. Again, similar results were not found for residents without ADRD. Given that previous studies have linked for-profit operating status, higher levels of onsite accidents, and greater incidence levels of decubiti with poorer nursing home quality-of-care practices, these findings raise some interesting questions about the motivation for hospitalizing nursing home residents with ADRD. For example, it may be that for-profit homes are more likely to transfer residents who are difficult to care for or who might pose certain liabilities. Thus, when a medical situation arises that contains higher levels of professional discretion in deciding whether or not to hospitalize, for-profit nursing homes may be more likely to hospitalize certain residents in order to minimize losses. Alternatively, it may be that these types of quality-of-care-related complications are more likely to arise in for-profit facilities, as some research has suggested, and thus, the increased risk of high discretion hospitalizations may be the outcome of the higher prevalence of quality problems.

Lastly, although study findings indicated that nurse practitioners play important roles in reducing high discretion hospitalizations for all nursing home residents, the findings appear to be particularly notable for residents with ADRD, who may be less able to communicate medical needs and to participate fully in decisions regarding their own care (Porell & Carter, 2005). These findings highlight important implications of ongoing public policy debates taking place regarding adequate staffing levels and quality-of-care practices in nursing homes for residents with ADRD. While much of the ongoing debate has tended to focus on the importance of increasing unlicensed personnel (e.g., Stone & Wiener, 2001) in general, the preceding discussion underscores not only the need for increased licensed nursing staff in particular; it also points to the pivotal role of licensed nursing staff in caring for nursing home residents with ADRD. In other words, the optimal management of ADRD so as to maintain a nursing home resident's quality of life is a challenge that involves a mix of interrelated social, medical, and behavioral inputs (Volicer, 2001). A trained licensed nursing staff plays an important role not only in the regular delivery of high quality care to nursing home residents, but also in the effective interfacing of this care with other components of the larger medical care system.

From a public policy standpoint, consideration of the study findings to date, coupled with the growing body of literature underscoring the important role of professionally licensed nursing staff in caring for frail elders, suggests that targeting chronic conditions for best care practices in the nursing home will assist efforts to reduce unnecessary hospitalizations. Most residents of nursing homes have multiple ongoing medical needs. Residents with both Alzheimer's disease and diabetes, for example, would likely benefit from improved daily ambulatory care practices in the nursing home. Programs targeted to these residents might include awareness training for nursing assistants, improved nutritional care planning and monitoring for residents, more frequent blood glucose screenings, and skin conditioning programs to prevent necrotic breakdown, to name a few. Although important for all residents, adequate knowledge, expertise, and professional staffing are crucial for residents with ADRD due to their inability to draw attention to their own immediate healthcare needs.

SEARCHING FOR APPROPRIATE HOSPITALIZATION RATES

Although complicated in nature, the unique characteristics of how nursing homes are structured and how they operate are important determinants of hospital use. Moreover, residents with ADRD appear to be particularly vulnerable to the effects of organizational and structural attributes of the nursing home in which they reside. Because the system relied upon to provide medical assistance for optimal functioning actually contributes, at least in part, to the risk of unnecessary and/or preventable hospitalizations, a careful consideration of the current policies aimed at improving nursing home care is necessary. For example, more effort is needed to understand the effects of resident location within the larger health care system and how the interaction of the individual with the broader contextual arrangement affects hospitalization practices for nursing home residents with ADRD.

While the relative importance of nursing home operational and structural characteristics in determining hospital use among residents is somewhat troubling, more optimistically it does help identify areas for public policy to address over- and underutilization of hospital treatment among vulnerable nursing home residents, particularly with respect to developing best practice guidelines targeted to specific populations in the nursing home. Efforts in developing best practices for residents with ADRD should include care strategies that seek to minimize reliance on unfamiliar caregivers, to increase licensed personnel including RNs and nurse practitioners, and to implement early interventions at the first sign of challenging behaviors.

The ongoing policy struggle involves not only pinpointing inappropriate and unnecessary hospitalizations, but also identifying the system-level factors that lead to the inappropriate hospitalization, for example, insufficient monitoring of care, communication barriers, and discontinuity of care providers, and then altering the care environment. Continued effort to understand the role of facility- and market-level determinants of hospitalization should provide valuable insight regarding the salient connections between subacute and acute care, as well as assist in future efforts to identify appropriate hospitalization practices affecting vulnerable populations of nursing home residents.

REFERENCES

Bergman, H., & Clarfield, A. M. (1991). Appropriateness of patient transfer from a nursing home to an acute-care hospital: a study of emergency room visits and hospital admissions. *Journal of the American Geriatrics Society, 39*(12), 1164–1168.

Berlowitz, D. R., Brandeis, G. H., Anderson, J., & Brand, H. K. (1997). Predictors of pressure ulcer healing among long-term care residents. *Journal of the American Geriatrics Society, 45*(1), 30–34.

Bliesmer, M. M., Smayling, M., Kane, R. L., & Shannon, I. (1998). The relationship between nursing staffing levels and nursing home outcomes. *Journal of Aging and Health, 10*(3), 351–371.

Buchanan, R. J., Madel, R. P., & Persons, D. (1991). Medicaid payment policies for nursing home care: A national survey. *Health Care Financing Review, 13*(1), 55–72.

Burger, S. G., Kayser-Jones, J., & Bell, J. P. (2000). *Malnutrition and dehydration in nursing homes: Key issues in prevention and treatment.* (A Report to the Commonwealth Fund No. 386). New York: Commonwealth Fund.

Burton, L. C., German, P. S., Gruber-Baldini, A. L., Hebel, J. R., Zimmerman, S., & Magaziner, J. (2001). Medical care for nursing home residents: Differences by dementia status. Epidemiology of Dementia in Nursing Homes Research Group. *Journal of the American Geriatrics Society, 49*(2), 142–147.

Carter, M. W. (2003a). Factors associated with ambulatory care-sensitive hospitalizations among nursing home residents. *Journal of Aging and Health, 15*(2), 295–331.

Carter, M. W. (2003b). Variations in hospitalization rates among nursing home residents: the role of discretionary hospitalizations. *Health Services Research, 38*(4), 1177–1206.

Carter, M. W., & Porell, F. W. (2002). *The relationship between nursing home performance on quality indicators and resident risk of hospitalization.* Presented at the 55th Annual Meeting of the Gerontological Society of America, Boston.

Carter, M. W., & Porell, F. W. (2003). Variations in hospitalization rates among nursing home residents: The role of facility and market attributes. *The Gerontologist, 43*(2), 175–191.

Carter, M. W., & Porell, F. W. (2003b). *Potentially avoidable hospitalizations among nursing home residents: Comparing residents with and without Alzheimer's disease.* Annual Meeting of the Gerontological Society of America, San Diego, CA.

Castle, N., & Fogel, B. (1998). Characteristics of nursing homes that are restraint free. *The Gerontologist, 38*(2), 181–188.

Castle, N. G., & Mor, V. (1996). Hospitalization of nursing home residents: A review of the literature, 1980–1995. *Medical Care Research and Review, 53*(2), 123–148.

Coburn, A. F., Keith, R. G., & Bolda, E. J. (2002). The impact of rural residence on multiple hospitalizations in nursing facility residents. *The Gerontologist, 42*(5), 661–666.

Creditor, M. C. (1993). Hazards of hospitalization of the elderly. *Annals of Internal Medicine, 118*(3), 219–223.

Dey, A. N. (1997). *Characteristics of elderly nursing home current residents: Data from the 1995 National Nursing Home Survey.* (Advance data from vital and health statistics No. 289). Hyattsville, MD: National Center for Health Statistics.

Evans, D. A. (1996). Descriptive epidemiology of Alzheimer's disease. In Z. S. Khachaturian, and T. S. Radebaugh (Eds.), *Alzheimer's disease: Causes, diagnosis, treatment, and care* (pp. 51–60). Boca Raton, FL: CRC Press, pp. 51–60.

Fabiszewski, K. J., Volicer, B., & Volicer, L. (1990). Effect of antibiotic treatment on outcome of fevers in institutionalized Alzheimer patients. *Journal of the American Medical Association, 263*(23), 3168–3172.

Fillenbaum, G., Heyman, A., Peterson, B. L., Pieper, C. F., & Weiman, A. L. (2001). Use and cost of hospitalization of patients with AD by stage and living arrangement: CERAD XXI. *Neurology, 56*(2), 201–206.

Freiman, M. P., & Murtaugh, C. M. (1993). The determinants of the hospitalization of nursing home residents. *Journal of Health Economics, 12*(3), 349–359.

Freiman, M. P., & Murtaugh, C. M. (1995). Interactions between hospital and nursing home use. *Public Health Reports, 110*(5), 546–554.

Fried, T. R., & Mor, V. (1997). Frailty and hospitalization of long-term stay nursing home residents. *Journal of the American Geriatrics Society, 45*(3), 265–269.

Gabrel, C. S. (2000a). *An overview of nursing home facilities: Data from the 1997 National Nursing Home Survey.* (Advance data from vital and health statistics No. 311). Hyattsville, MD: National Center for Health Statistics.

Gabrel, C. S. (2000b). *Characteristics of elderly nursing home current residents and discharges: Data from the 1997 National Nursing Home Survey.* (Advance data from vital and health statistics No. 312). Hyattsville, MD: National Center for Health Statistics.

Harrington, C., Zimmerman, D., Karon, S. L., Robinson, J., & Beutel, P. (2000). Nursing home staffing and its relationship to deficiencies. *The Journals of Gerontology Series B, Psychological Sciences and Social Sciences, 55*(5), S278–287.

Holtzman, J., & Lurie, N. (1996). Causes of increasing mortality in a nursing home population. *Journal of the American Geriatrics Society, 44*(3), 258–264.

Intrator, O., Castle, N. G., & Mor, V. (1999). Facility characteristics associated with hospitalization of nursing home residents: results of a national study. *Medical Care, 37*(3), 228–237.

Kayser-Jones, J. S., Wiener, C. L., & Barbaccia, J. C. (1989). Factors contributing to the hospitalization of nursing home residents. *The Gerontologist, 29*(4), 502–510.

Liu, K., Wissoker, D., & Rimes, C. (1998). Determinants and costs of Medicare post-acute care provided by SNFs and HHAs. *Inquiry, 35*(1), 49–61.

Mor, V., Intrator, O., Brandt, E., Fries, B. E., Phillips, C., & Teno, J., et al. (1997). Changes in hospitalization associated with introducing the Resident Assessment Instrument. *Journal of the American Geriatrics Society, 45*(8), 1002–1010.

Murtaugh, C. M., & Freiman, M. P. (1995). Nursing home residents at risk of hospitalization and the characteristics of their hospital stays. *The Gerontologist, 35*(1), 35–43.

Ouslander, J. G. (1988). Reducing the hospitalization of nursing home residents. *Journal of the American Geriatrics Society, 36*(2), 171–173.

Porell, F. W., & Carter, M. W. (2005). Discretionary hospitalization of nursing home residents with and without Alzheimer's disease: A multilevel analysis. *Journal of Aging and Health 17*(2), 207–230.

Rhoades, J., Potter, D. E. B., & Krauss, N. (1998). *Nursing homes: Structure and selected characteristics, 1996.* Rockville, MD: Agency for Healthcare Quality Research. MEP Research Findings No. 4. AHCPR Pub. No. 98–0006.

Roos, N. P., Wennberg, J. E., & McPherson, K. (1988). Using diagnosis-related groups for studying variations in hospital admissions. *Health Care Financing Review, 9*(4), 53–62.

Rubenstein, L. Z., Josephson, K. R., & Osterweil, D. (1996). Falls and fall prevention in the nursing home. *Clinics in Geriatric Medicine, 12*(4), 881–902.

Rubenstein, L. Z., Ouslander, J. G., & Wieland, D. (1988). Dynamics and clinical implications of the nursing home-hospital interface. *Clinical Geriatric Medicine, 4*(3), 471–491.

Sloss, E. M., Solomon, D. H., Shekelle, P. G., Young, R. T., Saliba, D., & MacLean, C. H., et al. (2000). Selecting target conditions for quality of care improvement in vulnerable older adults. *Journal of the American Geriatrics Society, 48*(4), 363–369.

Spector, W. D., Fleishman, J. A., Pezzin, L. E., & Spillman, B. C. (2000). *The characteristics of long-term care users.* A report to the Committee on Improving Quality in Long-Term Care, Institute of Medicine. Agency for Healthcare Research and Quality (AHRQ) Research Report. AHRQ Publication No. 00–0049.

Spector, W. D., & Takada, H. A. (1991). Characteristics of nursing homes that affect resident outcomes. *Journal of Aging and Health, 3*(4), 427–454.

Stone, R. I., & Wiener, J. M. (2001). *Who will care for us? Addressing the long-term care workforce crisis.* A report to the Office of Disability, Aging, and Long-Term Care Policy, Office of the Assistant Secretary for Planning and

Evaluation, U. S. Department of Health and Human Services. Washington, DC: Robert Wood Johnson Foundation.

Sullivan-Mark, E. M., Strumpf, N. E., Evans, L. K., Baumgarten, M., & Maislin, G. (1999). Predictors of continued physical restraint use in nursing home residents following restraint reduction efforts. *Journal of the American Geriatrics Society, 47*(3), 342–348.

Teresi, J. A., Holmes, D., Bloom, H. G., Monaco, C., & Rosen, S. (1991). Factors differentiating hospital transfers from long-term care facilities with high and low transfer rates. *The Gerontologist, 31*(6), 795–806.

Volicer, L. (2001). Management of severe Alzheimer's disease and end-of-life issues. *Clinics in Geriatric Medicine, 17(2)*, 377–391.

Volicer, L., & Hurley, A.C. (1997). Physical status and complications in patients with Alzheimer's disease: Implications for outcome studies. *Alzheimer's Disease and Associated Disorders, 11*, 60–65.

Wennberg, J. E., Barnes, B. A., & Zubkoff, M. (1982). Professional uncertainty and the problem of supplier-induced demand. *Social Science and Medicine, 16*(7), 811–824.

Won, A., Lapane, K., Gambassi, G., Bernabei, R., Mor, V., & Lipsitz. (1999). Correlates and management of nonmalignant pain in the nursing home. *Journal of the American Geriatrics Society, 47*(8), 936–942.

Zimmerman, S., Gruber-Baldini, A. L., Hebel, J. R., Sloane, P. D., & Magaziner, J. (2002). Nursing home facility risk factors for infection and hospitalization: importance of registered nurse turnover, administration, and social factors. *Journal of the American Geriatrics Society, 50*(12), 1987–1995.

PART II

Four Perspectives on the Hospital Experience for Persons with Dementia

CHAPTER FOUR

The Hospital Experience

Perspectives of Assisted Living Providers

Joan Hyde

Current surveys of assisted living residences report that between 30% and 50% of residents have some levels of cognitive impairment (ALFA, 2000; GAO, 1999; Hawes, Rosen, & Phillips, 1999; Hyde, 1995). One reason people move to assisted living settings is to get personalized oversight and coordination of their care needs, including coordination of care when they need hospitalization. This type of service would seem to be particularly important to those with cognitive impairment.

As cited in other chapters in this volume, individuals with dementia are particularly vulnerable to the problems all patients encounter in hospitals. This chapter reports on a small pilot study of hospitalizations among cognitively impaired residents living in six different assisted living communities. We conclude that assisted living can, if organized appropriately, provide coordination and support for resident transitions to the hospital and back to the assisted living facility, and thereby help reduce some of the problems with this aspect of a resident's hospital experience.

DESCRIPTION OF THE STUDY AND
THE STUDY POPULATION

Data were collected from interviews with a convenience sample of six nurses from assisted living residences in two states over a very limited time period (one month) in late 2003 (Table 4.1). Four of the facilities specialize in dementia care, and two serve a general assisted living population, including some cognitively impaired residents.

Based on this small sample (N = 318 residents with dementia), we found that an average of about 7% of assisted living residents were seen in a hospital emergency room (ER) over a given one-month period, and about 3% were admitted and spent one or more nights in the hospital, whether following an ER visit or as a planned admission. For the traditional assisted living residences in the sample, the staff was unable to break out the data for their cognitively impaired residents, so these numbers are for the mixed population. There is no significant difference in rates of ER use or hospitalizations between these two traditional assisted living residences and the four dementia-specific assisted living units.

Most of the hospitalizations experienced by cognitively impaired assisted living residents are for medical problems unrelated to their dementia. Hospitalizations for the behavioral and psychological symptoms of dementia are typically in a psychiatric hospital or the psychiatric wing of a general hospital. These psychiatric admissions are different in many ways from ER or acute hospital admissions, and their differing issues are outside the purview of this chapter.

Falls, fractures, and stroke were the main reasons reported for ER visits and/or hospitalizations. Table 4.2 illustrates the range and frequency of the conditions that were reported.

TABLE 4.1 Emergency Room Usage and Hospital Admissions (Monthly Averages, by Assisted Living Residence)

Facility code	Number of residents	Number of emergency room trips	ER trips/ number of residents (%)	Number of hospital admissions	Hospital admission (%)
Traditional A	90	8	9	2	2
Traditional B	95	4	4	3	3
SCU C	50	2	4	1	2
SCU D	26	1	4	2	8
SCU E	28	4	14	2	7
SCU F	29	2	7	0	0
Total/Average	318	21	7	10	3

Note: Data were reported by sites based on their last reporting period during the fall of 2003. The precise reporting period varied by site, and a one-month average obtained if the reporting period exceeded one month.

TABLE 4.2   Conditions Triggering an ER Visit or Hospitalization (in Order of Frequency)

Condition	Approximate % (N = 31)
Falls or fractures (other than hip)	25
Hip fracture	20
Strokes, chest pains, blood pressure changes	20
Pneumonia, urinary tract or other infection	15
Changes in mental status, behaviors	10
Other	10

CONCERNS OF ASSISTED LIVING STAFF ABOUT HOSPITALIZATION

In this brief survey, we heard reports of many of the same kinds of problems described in other chapters of this volume that are likely to occur when any person with dementia goes to the hospital. The following quotation from an assisted living staff person illustrates the frustration:

> "We've had people in the ER for 6, 7, 8 hours, and they don't even do anything . . . at least they should admit them into a room so they have a place to wait. They don't understand what's involved with the process of handling dementia patients and they'll ask the resident questions about medical history, which the patient can't answer. They ask the resident, have you had any surgery? And the resident looks at them like they've got 4 heads."

Some hospital staff, despite being told that the patient has dementia and despite witnessing the patient's inability to respond, nonetheless continue to expect the patient to report both recent and longer term medical and social history, even family members' telephone numbers.

Waiting areas are also problematic. Some ERs have people with dementia waiting on stretchers in busy hallways and fail to provide hydration, assistance with toileting, or other basic needs during long waits. They may not even have briefs available for incontinent patients who are spending many hours in the ER. An assisted living staff member underscores the need to accompany the cognitively impaired elder:

> "We think no older persons should go to the ER by themselves because they will be totally confused and traumatized. If they need help or if they have to go to the bathroom, they don't even know how to tell anybody. And in the ER, people wait hours unless they are having

a heart attack or something like that. For all these reasons, someone needs to accompany them."

Some hospitals have no system for evaluating and monitoring residents who are at risk for wandering out of the building or becoming lost, with no security systems to prevent wandering within or out of the building.

Moreover, many hospital staff members are unfamiliar with the behavioral symptoms of dementia and do not effectively prevent or deal with agitation and other psycho-behavioral symptoms that patients often display under the combined stresses of acute illness and hospitalization. Some ER staff members expect the patient to identify the assisted living staff member who accompanied the patient before they will allow the staff member to stay with the patient.

Residents who spend more than a day or two in the hospital often show signs of having been restrained, such as bed sores and loss of the ability to walk. The failure to order physical therapy or other interventions that would benefit a patient, either while in the hospital or as part of the follow-up plan, simply because the patient has dementia contributes to poorer outcomes following discharge.

CHALLENGES FOR THE ASSISTED LIVING PROVIDER

There are some specific problems that assisted living providers encounter when their residents go to the hospital. For example, families may not understand that assisted living providers must call 911 in an emergency, even when there is a standing Do Not Resuscitate order.

Ambulance companies and the local hospitals have agreements regarding to which hospital the ambulance will take someone. While in a life-threatening emergency it makes sense to take a patient to the nearest hospital, in other cases it would be better to take the patient to the hospital where his or her doctor is on staff or where the assisted living provider has established a good working relationship. Because these individuals live in assisted living residences and cannot speak for themselves, and because the staff cannot always reach a family member quickly enough, assisted living providers may have trouble advocating (and guaranteeing payment for) a transfer to the hospital of choice.

Further, some hospital staff do not understand that assisted living venues have different rules and capabilities from nursing homes, and they therefore assume that they can return a patient to his or her assisted living residence and the patient will get the same services as if he or she were returning to a nursing home.

"We've had people call up and say they're going to discharge someone, and the resident is just not in a condition to come back. The [hospital staff] doesn't understand under what conditions we can accept someone back. They don't know that we can't accept people with catheters – that's happened two times, almost three times. They're also not accommodating when it comes to discharge timings. They wanted to discharge someone at night; they were pushing to discharge this resident at 7 p.m. on Friday, but we wanted them to discharge the resident at a different time because we didn't have a nurse present at that time."

Conversely, the hospital staff may believe that since the patient comes from an assisted living residence, he or she must not have dementia. Or once they realize that the patient has dementia, staff members may assume that the patient cannot return to the assisted living residence and automatically refer the patient to a nursing home.

There is a lack of understanding of what the particular assisted living personnel can or cannot do. For example, in many states (Hyde, 1995), assisted living nurses cannot take orders for medication over the phone, and most assisted living residences cannot manage catheters and IVs. Also, hospital staff members often do not realize that assisted living residences generally do not have a nurse on site 24 hours a day.

Paperwork sent to the hospital, including the original "do not resuscitate" forms, often gets lost or is filed at the hospital, requiring assisted living staff either to retrieve or reestablish the paperwork.

Hospitals and ERs may discharge a patient without notice or without an adequate plan, and with little or no communication between hospital staff and assisted living staff, sometimes occasioned by privacy concerns.

HOW ASSISTED LIVING PROVIDERS CAN HELP REDUCE PROBLEMS FOR RESIDENTS WITH DEMENTIA WHO MUST GO TO THE HOSPITAL

Some assisted living residences surveyed for this study had better experiences than others with their local hospitals. While some of the difference is undoubtedly the result of better systems and training within the hospitals, some assisted living providers have taken steps that have improved residents' hospital experiences and that better serve their residents following the hospitalization:

1. *Accompany a person with dementia to the emergency room.* If a family member is not available to ride in the ambulance or meet the resident in the ER, a staff member should go with the patient and stay

until family arrives. For this strategy to be effective, the staff person must be reasonably fluent in English, knowledgeable about hospital systems, and willing to act as an advocate, which may mean that the staff member should be a nurse or other manager. Typically, assisted living residences that provide this service charge the families for it at a rate that covers the additional staff time. Even when paid for by families, it may be difficult for the assisted living residence to make a staff person available on an unplanned basis. An assisted living staff member describes the importance of accompanying the elder in the ER:

> "When one of our resident[s] goes to the ER, we find that many ER staff members do not understand that the resident has Alzheimer's, and they think they can just talk to him or her in a loud voice. The resident becomes agitated, and sometimes the doctor just leaves the resident there to wait. This situation has happened quite a few times. Now, an aide or a manager accompanies a resident; otherwise, the resident may be left in the ER for hours."

2. *Work with the local ambulance services.* Doing so can ensure that ambulance personnel understand the needs of those they are transporting and that they understand the assisted living provider's systems, as well as the importance of transmitting the paperwork given to them for use at the hospital. This work is ongoing, as illustrated by the following quotation:

> "Our paperwork that we send with the residents either gets lost in the ER or never gets to the ER. The ambulance company blames it on the ER and vice versa. So here we are trying to make their lives easier by giving med sheets, and yet they tend to lose them."

3. *Provide a clear summary of the resident's diagnosis and history.* Further, include a medication record, description of pre-emergency dementia symptoms, and phone numbers for next of kin. Include a copy of insurance information and the health care proxy document if one exists; send this information with the resident in the ambulance. If available, be sure to provide an acceptable copy of the DNR document as well. It takes considerable prior planning to ensure that accurate, up-to-date information is available, even during the night, if someone goes to the hospital on an emergency basis. That information is described by the following quotation:

> "We send a [specific, prearranged nursing home] authorization along with each resident, that should the resident need rehab, he or she will go to that nursing home, and the residence gets med sheet with the diagnosis, medication information, physician's and family's names and

numbers, and medical cards. We send two copies, one for hospital and one for ambulance people; yet, invariably, the hospital calls and says 'what meds is this person on' or 'what's the person's contact number.'"

4. *An assisted living nurse should call the ER while the resident is in transit.* The assisted living nurse must talk directly to the intake nurse, giving the intake nurse a medical history of the patient. The nurse should brief the ER on the need to have an assisted living staff member stay with the patient and give the name of the staff member accompanying the resident. Make sure the intake department knows how to reach both the assisted living nursing staff and the family.

5. *Arrange for private-duty aide.* If the resident is admitted to the hospital and is likely to have behavioral issues or need more assistance with activities of daily living (ADLs) than the hospital can provide, staff members should work with the family and the hospital to arrange for a private-duty aide.

6. *Prepare the assisted living staff for the resident's return.* Make sure that assisted living staff members who will be providing assistance know about any new medications or written instructions from the ER.

WORKING WITH HOSPITALS BETWEEN CRISES AROUND RESIDENT TRANSFERS

The intervention that assisted living staff members have found to be most helpful is creating and maintaining relationships with the hospital at times when there is no crisis. This requires:

- Visiting the hospital to understand its systems
- Dropping off materials about the assisted living facility
- Inviting key hospital staff to visit the assisted living residence so they have first-hand understanding of the residents when not in crisis and have an understanding of the assisted living facility
- Providing in-service training to hospital staff on dementia, including strategies for averting and managing wandering, agitation, and other behavioral issues

CONCLUSION

Assisted living staff members have considerable experience with the needs of people with dementia as they move through the hospital system. Staff members are an effective resource to work with other groups, such as the Alzheimer's Association, to help educate hospital staff about the needs of patients with dementia.

Assisted living residents are fortunate in that they often have both family members and assisted living staff acting as advocates. Consequently, assisted living residents with dementia may fare better than some cognitively impaired elders in the community who may have less support when they need to go to the hospital. Nonetheless, hospitalization continues to be an issue for this subset of the dementia population.

REFERENCES

Assisted Living Federation of America. (2000). *ALFA's overview of the assisted living industry*. Annapolis, MD: National Investment Center.

General Accounting Office. (1999). *Assisted living: Quality-of-care and consumer protection issues in four states*. Washington, DC: U.S. Congress/GAO.

Hawes, C., Rose, M., & Phillips, C. (1999). *National study of assisted living for the frail elderly*. Washington, DC: U.S. DHHS, ASPE.

Hyde, J. (1995). *Serving people with dementia: Regulating assisted living and residential care settings*. Lexington, MA: Hearthstone Press.

A Geriatric Social Worker's Perspective on Alzheimer's Patients in the Emergency Room

Sonia Michelson

An Alzheimer's patient in the emergency room is vulnerable to a rapid escalation of risks. The fundamental problem is twofold: (1) Alzheimer's disease rarely requires emergency care; however, the presence of Alzheimer's disease may impact on treatment for an emergency medical condition that is distinct from the Alzheimer's. (2) Current practice is not structured to recognize dementia as an operating factor in the patient's presenting problem.

Many factors contribute to the particular risks for Alzheimer's patients in the emergency room. The compromised mental status of the patient combined with a sudden urgent medical problem creates a diagnostic and treatment challenge for the brisk environment of emergency care. Clouds of the patient's confusion, a dilemma for which the fast-paced emergency room does not always have the necessary time or patience, may obscure the seriousness of the patient's medical problems. For elderly patients, and particularly for Alzheimer's patients, the emergency room can be a poor fit as slowly revealed information becomes entangled with rapidly moving actions. While well-intentioned medical personnel may attempt and give emergency care, there can be a formidable communications gap between patient and practitioners, as well as extraordinary stress for the patient. In the absence of information, medical staff may wonder about the purpose or need for emergency care.

Background

The author of this chapter is a social worker and geriatric care manager providing care for elderly clients who live in a variety of settings from independent living in their own homes to assisted living and long-term care facilities. Many of these clients have Alzheimer's disease, and most are fragile due to mental and physical impairments. Within this population, it is not unusual for people to experience a variety of medical events including acute and life-threatening illness. In the absence of a medical practitioner or necessary diagnostic equipment, medical assessment is difficult and fraught with the risks of missing a serious problem.

Emergency room care may begin with the perception of a problem as it is observed and understood by the caregiver rather than a patient's statement or display of specific symptoms. When a family member or assisted living staff member observes an elder with sudden or significant changes in behavior, the emergency room may become the destination for care, especially if the primary care provider is not immediately available or accessible.

The following vignettes of Anna, a fictitious client, are based on the author's experiences and represent a composite of emergency room situations encountered over years of working with Alzheimer's patients. The vignettes describing five hours of emergency room waiting and treatment highlight the particular and continuing risks for Alzheimer's patients encountering a new and complex environment. Anna's risks through emergency care were mitigated by the presence and advocacy of an informed caregiver; however, for an unaccompanied patient, there is typically no patient advocate on site. For patients who are accompanied by a family member or other caregiver, constant and vigilant attention is essential.

ANNA

This vignette describes a 90-year old female client who resided in an assisted living facility. Anna had moved from her two-family home when both home and health management declined precipitously due to advancing Alzheimer's disease. Anna lived on the "traditional" side of the facility because the staff felt that she could still manage well enough without the restrictions of the dementia unit. Her social skills remained very much intact; in fact, her smile, easy laugh, and remarkable agility made her a favorite among residents and staff.

Anna had been in the assisted living facility for about six months when I received a call late on a Friday afternoon. "Anna needs medical attention before the weekend," said the nurse. "She has a prolapsed something and she is having a lot of distress. If she is not seen before the weekend, I am concerned that she will get worse. And you know, Anna is not a complainer. She should go to the emergency room."

This call of reported distress points out some systemic tangles that impact emergency care. As a social worker and care manager, my responsibility is to address the range of needs in the lives of my clients, and in this situation, to provide relief and prevent a worsening crisis. I do not make medical assessments and depend on medical practitioners to provide the information that dictates treatment. In this situation, I knew that the nurse's reports could only be based on Anna's verbal complaints, since state regulations limit the role of assisted living personnel in providing medical assessments.

While patients utilizing emergency rooms have certain common experiences, there are identifiable differences for Alzheimer's patients. Following are some of the major problems confronting most emergency room patients as well as identification of additional risks for Alzheimer's patients:

1. **Urgent need for care.** There is an unexpected and urgent medical problem requiring immediate attention. The medical problem is usually perceived by the patient who can articulate the complaint well enough and express or demonstrate the need for care.
   Differences for the Alzheimer's Patient: The matter of urgency may be driven as much by the concern of a caregiver who may or may not know the patient well and who may not accompany the patient to the hospital. The Alzheimer's patient may have lost the ability to understand or report sensations of bodily change or illness. In addition, the patient's language decrements may be confusing to the caregiver, who in turn may feel heightened concern and need for medical intervention.

2. **Diagnosis for elderly patients is complex and often subtle.** Without training in geriatric medicine, emergency room personnel may have limited experience in identifying potentially serious medical problems in older patients.
   Differences for the Alzheimer's Patient: When information is limited by patient reporting, many extra diagnostic tests may be

ordered to avoid risk of an adverse reaction to treatment. Care may also include verbal rather than written follow-up instructions that may not be remembered, particularly if told in the absence of a caregiver or patient advocate.

3. **Emergency care is often needed during the night and on weekends.** The medical problem becomes evident or causes concern when the primary care physician's office is closed.

    Differences for the Alzheimer's Patient: In the emergency room, patient and physician are likely to be meeting for the first time. While emergency physicians are trained for efficient diagnosis and treatment, both patient and practitioner have additional challenges when they have their first encounter in the emergency room. For the patient, meeting an unfamiliar practitioner in an unfamiliar and confusing setting may add to the patient's feelings of distress and further compound the challenges of communication and diagnosis. In addition, patients with early to moderate Alzheimer's disease have other risks. With better-preserved social skills and command of language, their apparent unremarkable behavior and language may mask both the Alzheimer's disease as well as an emerging medical condition.

4. **Absence of medical records.** Emergency room personnel may not have access to the patient's medical records. The reliability of patient reporting is variable.

    Differences for the Alzheimer's Patient: Because emergency room care may not be given in a hospital where the patient has previously received care, important history may not be available at the time of an emergency admission. A medical record would likely carry the presence of dementia, information that could help to guide the course of medical care. Emergency room practitioners may not know if the patient is supplying reliable information, particularly when the patient appears to be competent and offers information that may appear plausible, even if incorrect.

5. **Patient fatigue.** Both waiting for and receiving treatment can take many hours. For patients whose conditions are determined to be less urgent, waiting room time is extensive.

    Differences for the Alzheimer's Patient: Alzheimer's patients are likely to be elderly and generally less robust than most people seeking emergency care. Long waits in the emergency room can be exhausting, overwhelming, and arduous for anyone, and even more so when the environment is unfamiliar and confusing. Physical and emotional discomfort escalates with long waits in hard chairs, and sometimes a shortage of seating space. Waiting time may also mean an absence of meals and possibly regular medications that are fundamental for well-being.

Back to Anna

In the absence of a clinical evaluation, the nurse was faced with a dilemma. Accepting Anna's expression of distress as a need for immediate care meant use of the emergency room as a safety net against a worsening condition. Although the severity of the complaint was difficult to assess, the nurse who knew Anna perceived that her patient's medical condition could escalate and create a more serious situation.

Immediate Risks for Anna:

- Caregiver challenged in assessing the complaint of the memory-impaired person
- Primary care physician not available
- Limited options for treatment
- Dementia not immediately obvious

Anna's Alzheimer's disease was moderate. In a first and hurried emergency room encounter, a patient like Anna could easily be perceived as high functioning because the presence of her dementia is obscured. While Anna's social skills and language were well preserved, her memory and ability to report accurately were severely compromised. She was likeable, charming, uncomplaining, and unlikely to remember that she had earlier presented herself to the nurse with signs of a prolapsed uterus. In the emergency room, she would be unlikely to report the symptoms that had caused her distress and worried the nurse.

Perception of Urgent Need for Medical Care

While Anna's complaints concerned the nurse, it was of equal concern that the problem was presented on a Friday afternoon when physician's offices are shutting down. Since assisted living facilities do not offer medical care, how could Anna be treated over the weekend if her discomfort escalated?

Considering the Options

With the weekend moving closer, I knew no doctor's office would be open to see her that day. Her physician was away and I spoke with the covering doctor for a recommendation. He concurred that it was too late to see a gynecologist, regretted that there was little that he could do, and agreed that the best option would be to go to the emergency room.

I could foresee a long evening in the emergency room and one that would not be easy for a 90-year-old woman whose medical needs would not rise to the top of triage priorities. She would be ranked as less urgent than the inevitable ambulance cases, accidents, and severe illnesses that flood emergency rooms with pain and fear, especially on Friday nights. It was with some misgivings that I picked up Anna at her assisted living facility and proceeded to the hospital, arriving about 5 p.m. on a cold and snowy evening. What followed for the next four hours represents a sampling of some of the challenges encountered in the emergency room by patients with Alzheimer's disease.

THE JOURNEY CONTINUES—
ARRIVING AT THE HOSPITAL

Parking the car was the first challenge. The emergency room parking lot was filled, necessitating taking the car to the hospital garage, a distance too far for Anna to manage in icy conditions. The waiting room was very busy and I could not see anyone to sit with her during my absence. Knowing Anna, I felt that she would not panic during my brief absence, so I found her a seat and prayed that my silent predictions of her behavior would prove true. I was relieved to find Anna where I left her when I returned from parking the car.

The next step was registration. I brought Anna to the registration desk where there was a straightforward interview with a hospital clerk. Anna was able to provide her name and date of birth accurately, and that was all. We were then told to wait for the triage nurse. "It will be just a few minutes," said the clerk. Anna and I found two seats, by then precious commodities in the quickly filling waiting room. When the triage nurse called Anna's name about 30 minutes later, Anna did not respond. It was possible that she did not hear the nurse's voice calling her name or that she was starting to feel fatigued, and possibly overwhelmed by the atmosphere in the room.

> *Immediate Risks for Anna:*
>
> - Absence of a safe arrival point
> - Absence of comfortable and secure seating
> - No identification of dementia problems

Emergency room design and practice assume that patients can enter the facility, follow instructions, and adapt to the procedures. For the most part, this is true, and for patients who are cognitively intact, the experience is endurable, albeit not pleasurable. The Alzheimer's patient is expected to conform and respond to the same visual and spoken directions and navigate through a new and unfamiliar world. Doorways, windows, and hallways have little meaning, and unfamiliar sounds and voices are irrelevant and possibly confusing when the emergency room has no context for the patient. The risks for wandering are ripe. Fatigue, hunger, and dehydration add to the mix, compounding the drain on stamina. For the Alzheimer's patient, the physical and emotional stressors are likely to lower mental status.

Why Are You Here? The Triage Experience

The triage nurse, a soft spoken and gentle man, asked Anna why she had come to the emergency room. "Well, I don't know," she said with her usual grace. "I think my pantyhose may have been too tight." The nurse flashed a puzzled look in my direction allowing me to clarify and briefly report on my earlier conversations with the assisted living staff. "I don't think it's anything," Anna continued. The nurse said we would need to wait for about an hour before seeing a doctor and that it would first be necessary to obtain a urine sample. He pointed in the direction of the bathroom and gave specific and detailed directions for collection of the specimen. Anna nodded in agreement, suggesting both understanding of the direction and intention of follow-through. However, when we left the room, Anna needed assistance to find the bathroom as well as specific help in following the instructions that she could not recall. I knew that this would be a long night for both of us, and once again, we found some unoccupied seats and settled in. My goal was to keep Anna comfortable and minimally stressed.

Anna could not remember or explain the reason for being in the emergency room. Her response to the nurse provided little information for diagnosis or treatment. Although she gave the impression of understanding the nurse's comments, she could not follow directions for her care. Without ongoing personal attention, Anna was again at risk for escalating confusion, wandering, and being lost in the maze of the fast-moving system. Additionally, as time passed, Anna was becoming more fatigued and in need of physical comfort and nourishment. We found some hard chairs that provided minimal comfort. The nearest food was in the hospital cafeteria, some distance away from the emergency room. I was reluctant to leave Anna because I was concerned about her potential for wandering or that she might be called and miss her turn.

The Wait Continues—More Decisions To Be Made

After one and a half hours had passed, the emergency room was becoming busier and the prospective waiting time loomed longer. I called the covering physician and asked his opinion about making a choice between waiting and bringing Anna home. "I really can't tell you," he replied. "I haven't seen her. If she is not complaining of pain at the moment, she may be okay." I then paged the nurse who had been certain about the urgent need for medical care. The nurse was no longer available; her assistant returned my call and said that the decision was mine to make. "You could bring her back to the assisted living," she said, "but if Anna has any further complaints of pain during the weekend, you will be called again."

The dilemma was to determine the best course of care for Anna. Was the wear of waiting in the emergency room better or worse than the chance of going home, being in pain, and not being able to access help during the night or weekend? I went back to speak with the triage nurse and said I was considering taking Anna home due to the long wait, now totaling two and a half hours. "Things are thinning out a bit and you may be next," he said. I promised that we would not leave without telling him.

Immediate Risks for Anna:

- Exhaustion
- Hunger
- Increased physical discomfort
- Agitation

As the evening progressed, the waiting in the crowded emergency room was taking its toll on Anna. Her fatigue was mounting, as was her discomfort from sitting in institutionally small and rigid chairs. I provided Anna with water to avoid dehydration; however, food was not nearby and I was reluctant to leave Anna or try to take her to the cafeteria. If I left her alone, she was at increasing risk for confusion and wandering in the hospital. In addition, she would not likely respond to her name being called, and consequently, would lose her place in the triage line. Anna's patience and good humor were also showing signs of wear from the cumulative effects of waiting. At this point, being in these circumstances made no sense to Anna. It was necessary and helpful to offer continuing reassurance, handholding, and distraction to support Anna through this period.

Medical Evaluation and Treatment

One hour later, we were called again and assigned a cubicle in the emergency room. This was the place where we would wait and eventually be seen by the doctor. Anna was given a hospital johnny and we were left alone. I helped Anna to undress and put on the johnny. About a half hour later, a nurse came into our cubicle and asked Anna to tell her why she had come to the emergency room. Anna's response remained essentially the same, that her pantyhose were the culprit to explain her malady. "Maybe I'm a little uncomfortable," she said.

When the doctor arrived, his questions were the same as the previous questions, and Anna continued to offer the same answers. Again, I offered an explanation that was respectful to Anna and could illuminate the diagnostic problem for the doctor. "We'll need to do an exam," he said. "I'll be back with a chaperone."

The bed was turned towards the wall, stirrups were placed, and Anna was helped to be in position for the exam. A few minutes passed and it was clear to me that Anna was uncomfortable. I requested that she not be kept in stirrups as she had previous hip surgery and the position was not comfortable for her. The nurse removed the stirrups and made a series of intermittent visits to the cubicle as we waited for the doctor to arrive. We kept up a distracting conversation for another half hour until the doctor returned.

The doctor performed a pelvic examination. "I don't see any evidence of a prolapse," he said. "She should follow-up with a gynecologist next week." We said our good-byes. I mentioned to the nurse that the patient had missed dinner and he immediately offered a box dinner for Anna to bring home. I helped Anna to get dressed and brought her back to the waiting room while I went to retrieve the car. We returned to the assisted living, rang the bell, and to Anna's surprise, the front door to her home was locked. An aide who knew Anna responded to the doorbell and admitted Anna to the building. At this point, Anna seemed relieved and comfortable in familiar surroundings. Anna and I bid each other good night, almost five hours after the beginning of our evening.

Although I informed each emergency room staff member of Anna's cognitive status, this information did not appear to be transmitted along the line of hospital personnel involved in her care. Anna was an unreliable reporter of her symptoms, and were it not for the presence of an advocate, her presence in the emergency room would likely have been more enigmatic.

Risks for Anna:
- Not identified as an Alzheimer's patient
- More waiting time
- Anna's inability to describe additional discomforts
- Transportation and safe return home
- Expectation for patient to follow-up on medical recommendations

---

The additional waiting time was likely due in part to a triage assessment of low urgency as well as the high level of activity in the emergency room. However, the Alzheimer's patient endures not only the discomfort of repeated portions of waiting, but also overall fatigue affect.

Anna did not speak out about discomforts during her care. Lying on a gurney surrounded by lights and technological equipment can be daunting to most patients. Anna had no memory of her prior hip surgery. That surgery, although successful, left her with some specific limitations in her mobility. She could not articulate either her additional distress or the reasons for it.

Anna's method for transportation home was evident. However, in the absence of another person, Anna might have traveled by taxi or possibly ambulance. Taxi transportation would have posed a variety of risks, including the wrong destination, potential difficulty of communicating with the driver, and difficulty with payment. An ambulance, while more reliable, would probably have felt overwhelming to the patient. In addition, ambulance transportation is costly and, in this situation, would have provided far more equipment and personnel than needed.

Recommendations for follow-up care are an expectable part of emergency care. However, in giving the recommendation, there is an implicit assumption that the recommendation can be followed. For the Alzheimer's patient, assumptions about compliance with follow-up instructions do not apply. While Anna nodded affirmatively to the recommendation, she would not remember hearing it, nor would she be able to follow the course of action.

FOLLOW-UP CARE

A week after the emergency room visit, I brought Anna to the gynecologist's office. From Anna's comments and the nurse's reports, there was no evidence that her physical complaints persisted. In addition, the events of the emergency room were no longer in Anna's memory. Her physical complaints had subsided. After I explained the reason for the visit, the doctor told Anna he would have to do a pelvic examination. As he was completing the examination, the doctor exclaimed, "A prolapse of the bladder and uterus. You can't miss it!" Anna listened with interest as the doctor explained the treatment options. By the time we left the office, that information had vanished from her memory.

Treatment decisions were ultimately made in consultation with Anna, her family who live at a distance, her physician, and me. I accompany Anna to the doctor's office for periodic follow-up visits and this arrangement allows for informed and appropriate care.

CONCLUSION

Why did the emergency room physician miss Anna's prolapsed uterus? Anna's experience highlights some of the identifiable systemic problems in emergency room care for Alzheimer's patients. For Anna, the hours in the emergency room were of little benefit to her, although of some relief to the assisted living staff. Although the emergency room physician did not see the medical problem, the prolapsed uterus, he did not discount a gynecological problem and made a referral to a specialist. Although the missed diagnosis may not have been directly attributable to Alzheimer's, it is possible that the physician did not have much experience in providing gynecological care for elderly women. Anna's inability to describe the problem may have further confounded the physician. Ultimately, one can only speculate about the reasons for the missed diagnosis.

Should Anna have gone to the emergency room? While hindsight makes it clear that Anna did not require emergency care, the confluence of weekend distress, the absence of a primary care physician, the regulatory prohibitions for assisted living personnel, and caregiver concern combined for action believed to be in Anna's best interest.

The emergency room culture is not well matched for older adults and particularly older adults with dementia. Given the growth of the elderly population and need for emergency medical care, two recommendations are offered that could enhance care and provide better outcomes:

1. An advocate for older adults on the emergency room staff with particular training in dementia could screen for dementia and could assist and support practitioners with communications. In addition, attention could be given to the particular risks for Alzheimer's patients.

2. Training should be provided for all emergency room personnel for better recognition of Alzheimer's and awareness of how the underlying condition may affect treatment of another presenting problem.

CHAPTER SIX

The Acute Care Experience in the Emergency Department

Mary Pat McKay, Susan Farrell, Khama Ennis, and
Emily Spilseth Binstadt

THE EMERGENCY DEPARTMENT EXPERIENCE

The Emergency Department (ED) is a singular environment. Just walking through the space is confusing and chaotic, with a horde of people busily doing many different jobs. And there are alarming sounds: beeps, whistles, ringing telephones, and sounds of people crying, vomiting, arguing, or simply talking. For one who becomes an ED patient, there is the discomfort of waiting with strangers, being uncovered, feeling too warm or too cool, and being asked to lie patiently on a hard, narrow stretcher. Few people are pleasantly excited about coming to the ED, coming only when something is wrong. Sometimes the issue is simple and the visit mostly an inconvenience, but many people who become ED patients fear the diagnosis and the potential pain associated with caring for a problem.

Being in the ED can be even more difficult for patients with dementia. Because of their cognitive problems, they are less able to cope with many different kinds of sensory input and less able to tolerate the apparently slow process of care. The difficulty begins in the waiting room where they meet and register with the triage nurse and administrative team and are then asked to wait in what is often an overcrowded, loud, chaotic space. Critically ill patients are evaluated immediately, but patients with nonemergent problems can wait more than six hours to be seen. Times spent in waiting rooms vary among hospitals and by time of day and day of the week. One system's published average is 56 minutes after registration (Lambe et al., 2002). Demented patients may have difficulty registering and being triaged; these tasks involve finding an insurance card, recalling details such as primary physician, and speaking to three or four different people.

Once in the body of the ED, demented patients will be cared for by another group of people that may include clerks, nurses, aides, respiratory or radiology technicians, and physicians. Many of these interactions are brief; patients may be asked the same questions repeatedly and then asked to perform some physical task quickly (sit up, lie down, move over here). Individually, these interactions can be pleasant, but the accumulated stress on the patients' cognitive functioning can easily lead to impatience and frustration. Between interactions, there may be hours of waiting. Published average ED length-of-stay periods range from under three hours to more than seven hours (Lammers, Roiger, Rice, Overton, & Cucos, 2003; Partovi, Nelson, Bryan, & Walsh, 2001). Patience beyond reasonableness may be required to cope with the experience.

There are many reasons for a demented person to visit the ED. The patient may have an injury, medical problems (unrelated to the dementia), or an issue related to the dementia itself. One of the biggest problems from the point of view of the ED provider caring for the patient is information. The caregivers do not know the person. What is he or she normally like? Is today's behavior typical? If the concern is a change in mental status, is it really acute, signaling a new and potentially serious problem, or has a family member simply become aware of a further decline in the chronic condition? What medications are actually being taken? What medical problems does the patient have? Given the problems with short-term memory, sometimes even the complaint or concern that brought the patient to the ED is unclear by the time he or she sees the physician. Lack of good information can result in unnecessary testing that can be painful and time consuming. At the same time, good information about the patient helps providers minimize stress for the patient and optimize the diagnostic and treatment processes — something as simple as knowing that the person hears only from the right ear can facilitate an entire ED visit.

A second theme of the ED visit for demented patients centers around decision-making. Slowly developing issues frequently come to a head in the event of an acute medical problem. When are patients no longer able to make decisions for themselves? Who should intervene? What are patients' preferences for interventions? Presentations to the ED center on an acute (often truly emergent) problem; the "right" level of intervention may be unclear. For instance, the mildly demented person living at home with family who develops pneumonia and breathing difficulty might want to be placed onto a ventilator and expect to recover and return home in a few days. However, the severely demented patient who is confined to bed in a nursing home and unable to speak or care for him- or herself might not want to be on a ventilator in the same situation. Similar issues arise when sudden kidney failure might require dialysis or when the patient needs emergency surgery. The ED is not the best place to begin conversations about decision-making; these discussions are best begun well in advance of the emergency situation. Nonetheless, these issues frequently require urgent responses from the ED staff.

To optimize the situation for the demented patient in the ED, there are steps patients, families, caregivers, and primary physicians can take before and during the ED stay. In addition, there are strategies that ED staff can use to help keep the patient comfortable and minimize frustration.

Using vignettes, the authors' personal experiences, and medical research, this chapter provides insights into the communication, actions, and issues that can improve the ED experience.

CASE STUDY: COMMUNITY DWELLER, MRS. E

Mrs. E has been complaining to her daughter, Janice, of pain in her "backside" for several days. Today, Janice noticed her mother limping and insisted on taking her to the emergency department. A few days ago, Mrs. E told Janice that she had slipped on the stairs, but now Mrs. E does not remember the incident. In the waiting room chair, Mrs. E cannot get comfortable, and becomes more and more irritable, insisting to Janice that they must leave immediately. Janice is relieved when Mrs. E's name is finally called.

After Janice and her mother respond to the call, the nurse informs Janice that she will have to remain in the waiting room while her mother "gets settled." In the treatment area, Mrs. E is quite relieved to be lying flat, and although she is delighted by each of the nice people who inquires about her health, she emphasizes a different minor health concern to each one. She is consistent in her contention that her overall health is excellent and is proud to be living in her own home at age 80. She says her daughter Janice lives nearby. She begins to search for her daughter's phone number among the many slips of paper in her purse. She thinks she may have a list of her medications somewhere in there, too.

Not until Dr. C asks her to walk does she acknowledge the pain in her back. Dr. C orders X-rays. Although there are no obvious fractures, Dr. C explains that the bones are very thin (from osteoporosis), and he is worried about an injury in her pelvis. He recommends two weeks of bed rest, and Mrs. E says, "Good, I was worried that I would have to stay in the hospital." She is cheerful, and thanks Dr. C for being such a good doctor. When Janice is allowed back to see her, Mrs. E explains that "nothing is broken — I can go home." Janice is relieved that her mother has not fractured her hip, but wants to speak with Dr. C herself.

Janice tells Dr. C that she does not believe that her mother is capable of caring for herself any longer. Janice says that Mrs. E is becoming increasingly forgetful; just last week she forgot about her dinner on the stove until the smoke alarm went off. Dr. C insists that Mrs. E has no injuries requiring emergent hospitalization, but offers Janice and Mrs. E a consultation with the social worker, who confirms Janice's impression that Mrs. E will not be able to maintain the bed rest treatment on her own at home. When the social worker mentions the option of hospital admission as a means to finding Mrs. E another place to stay, Mrs. E becomes distraught and panicked.

Dr. C attempts to talk with Mrs. E about her concerns. Mrs. E screams, "She wants me to go to that Greenhaven place, you know, one of those homes for half-dead old people? Both my sisters died there, and if I ever end up there while I still have two feet and a brain that will let me do it, I'll walk right out before they even have time to unpack my bags! When it's my time, I want to go like my husband did, at peace in his own home. What are they going to fix by putting me in the hospital or in a home? The only thing wrong with me is that I am old!"

Who Decides?

Mrs. E's situation is not rare (Naughton, Moran, Kadah, Heman-Ackah, & Longano, 1995). Dementia is a difficult disease because it slowly erodes adults' capacities to care for themselves and make independent decisions. Dementia progresses at different rates in different people and leaves those with dementia and their families to balance the preservation of independent lifestyle with the need for supervision to ensure safety. During an ED visit, family members may have preexisting concerns about the patient and may try to garner support from the medical staff to enforce their solutions for the resistant elderly patient. Thus, to preserve their autonomy, elders may try to hide their impairments in the ED. Emergency physicians often can treat the acute injury or illness more easily than they can address the underlying ethical question: Is it time to adjust the balance between this patient's safety and independence?

Answering this question requires knowledge of the patient's cognitive abilities, the functional limitations caused by the injury or illness, and the social supports available in the patient's current living environment. A physician with the time pressures of a busy ED may not be able to assess accurately all of these factors. ED physicians do not document dementia and delirium in many elderly ED patients, possibly because they do not recognize these patients' impairments during brief visits (Birrer, Singh, & Kumar,1999; Lewis, Miller, & Morley 1995; Hustey, Meldon, & Palmer, 2000).

Mrs. E's health care providers initially assumed that Mrs. E's history was complete and truthful because she appeared so pleasant and conversational. Had no more knowledgeable caregiver been available, she might have simply been discharged. A private conversation between provider and patient allows the provider to ask about feelings of safety and the possibility of abuse and gives the patient an opportunity to bring up confidential issues. No socioeconomic or racial boundaries predict elder abuse and neglect. High-risk characteristics for elder abuse include patients with advanced age, physical handicaps, social isolation, emotional or financial dependence, inadequate housing, and caretakers with substance abuse problems. Many of these same risk factors predict increased ED use in elderly patients (Shah, Rathouz, & Chin, 2001). Because of these issues, adult patients must be interviewed privately during their ED stays.

In an effort to minimize the chaos in overcrowded and busy EDs, some systems routinely request family members to remain in the waiting room. This allows an initial opportunity for a private interaction between the patient and physician and also allows the nursing staff to draw blood or start an intravenous line without disconcerting family members or caregivers. However, in the case of a demented patient, early contact with a knowledgeable family member or caregiver can expedite care. Removing patients with dementia from their regular caregivers for more than a few minutes may cause needless agitation and delay providers from acquiring pertinent medical information. It is important for caregivers to remain throughout the sometimes long ED stays. Often, when the familiar person leaves, the patient becomes more agitated and may even require chemical or physical restraints that would be unnecessary otherwise (Eriksson, 1999). Caregivers may also have concerns they want to discuss privately with the provider and there should be an opportunity for that type of conversation as well. By informing the ED staff about the patient's dementia, a caregiver can join the patient during the examination as well as have private conversations with providers. Most ED staff members are eager to have assistance coping with patients who have trouble managing the demands of the ED environment.

Accurate information about health problems and medications is crucial to optimizing the care of patients with cognitive deficits in the ED. Even in this computerized age, physicians in the ED may not have ready access to medical charts. Caregivers should carry a list that includes health issues, allergies, and current medications. This list should include any vitamins, over-the-counter medications, and herbal products used regularly by the patient. One example of such a list is presented in Figure 6.1. In many situations, use of a MedicAlert tag (http://www. medicalert.org) on a necklace, anklet, or bracelet can provide lifesaving medical and contact information. Safe Return™ tags (http://www.alz. org/ResourceCenter/Programs/SafeReturn.htm) with the patient's address and contact information can also expedite care.

With good historical information and after a physical exam, the ED physician reaches a "differential diagnosis" or list of problems that might be causing the symptoms. A series of tests is often ordered to identify the correct answer from the list of possibilities. In a busy ED, this process can take several hours. Patients may have to hold still while blood is drawn or an intravenous catheter placed. They may be moved to another area for an Xray or CAT scan, where they may be moved onto a table and then asked to hold still again. After the tests are taken, there is a wait for results. While waiting, caregivers and ED staff can work to make patients comfortable by ensuring that they get their medicines at the usual times, are offered a meal (if medically allowed, since some tests cannot be performed on full stomachs), and have an opportunity to move around the bed or sit in a chair if it makes them more comfortable. In Mrs. E's case, she was comfortable during most of her early ED stay.

Medical Decision-Making Capacity

Once the ED physician reaches an adequate understanding of the patient's medical and social situation, he or she recommends a care plan. For Mrs. E, this was where the conflict arose: Mrs. E and Janice disagreed about the best plan of care. As long as adult patients can understand and reflect upon these recommendations, they should make their own treatment decisions. The capacity to make decisions about medical issues may wax and wane. Problems such as electrolyte imbalances, urinary tract infections, and strokes can masquerade as psychiatric problems in the elderly. Pain, in particular, can aggravate patients' behavioral challenges. Elderly patients with impaired cognition typically receive less pain medication than their peers without cognitive impairments (Feldt, Ryden, & Miles, 1998). Treatment of an acute disease process can preserve patients' autonomy. Demented patients may reveal intact cognition

DATE _____

Name: Mrs M.

Address:

Phone:

Narrative: Mrs. M is 82. She lives in an assisted living apartment. Normally she can safely walk without assistance and makes all her own meals. She often forgets little things like the day of the week. She no longer drives and her family now takes care of her shopping, but she takes care of keeping herself and the apartment immaculate.

Pt is oriented to:

Self	_X_ always	___ sometimes forgets	___ seldom recalls	___ never
Year	___ always	_X_ sometimes forgets	___ seldom recalls	___ never
Season	_X_ always	___ sometimes forgets	___ seldom recalls	___ never
Month	___ always	_X_ sometimes forgets	___ seldom recalls	___ never
Location	_X_ always	___ sometimes forgets	___ seldom recalls	___ never
Day	___ always	_X_ sometimes forgets	___ seldom recalls	___ never
Time	___ always	_X_ sometimes forgets	___ seldom recalls	___ never

Recognizes family and caregivers:

      ___ always _X_ sometimes forgets ___ seldom recalls ___ never

Conversation:

  _X_ Speaks clearly and can complete a conversation

  ___ Speaks in sentences but will sometimes lose the idea of the conversation

  ___ Sometimes forgets the end of the sentence

  ___ Speaks only occasionally

  ___ Makes noises but does not speak

First Language: English

Walking:

  _X_ Walks without help

  ___ Uses a cane

  ___ Uses a walker

  ___ Wheelchair bound but transfers with assistance

  ___ Unable to transfer

  ___ Bed bound

Activities of daily living (showering, dressing, brushing teeth, using the bathroom):

  _X_ Independently

  ___ Needs to be reminded but then can accomplish tasks herself

  ___ Needs assistance with _____

Hearing: no hearing in the left ear

Sight: Has had cataract surgery; uses glasses only to read.

Medical Problems: Diabetes, High Blood Pressure, Alzheimer's disease, Deaf in the left ear.

Surgeries: Appendectomy, gall bladder surgery, left hip replacement.

Allergies: Sulfa causes a rash.

Medications:

  Glucophage 1000 mg in the morning and 500 mg in the afternoon

  Lisinopril 5 mg in the morning

  Aspirin 81 mg in the morning

Most Recent Vital Signs (when well): BP 132/76 HR 74 Oxygen Saturation 95%

Health Care Proxy: Daughter: Natalie M, 100 Elm St., Your Town, MA, 00000. Phone (888) 555-1234, cell (888) 555-4567.

Primary Physician: Dr Smith, (888) 555-9887

Preferred Hospital: Town Hospital

Long-Term Wishes: Mrs. M wants to maintain her independence as long as possible. If she could be reasonably expected to return to her current level of functioning, she would want to be resuscitated by whatever means necessary. If she were no longer able to do things for herself and required assistance to do most things, she would no longer want to be resuscitated. She cannot imagine wanting a feeding tube for any reason.

Specific Concerns: Mrs. M gets upset and frustrated when she can't hear well.

FIGURE 6.1 Current level of functioning.

after doctors recognize and treat their pain, or address hearing and vision problems (Sugarman, McCrory, & Hubal, 1998). *Medical decision-making capacity* is the term used to identify patients with the right to make their own decisions. To be judged as having medical decision-making capacity, patients must want to make the decision and demonstrate the following capabilities:

1. Understand his/her medical status, the proposed interventions or procedures, and the alternative treatment options.
2. Comprehend the likely consequences, risks, and benefits of various treatment options, including no intervention.
3. Make a voluntary and reproducible choice by referencing personal values, goals, and wishes.
4. Describe a "chain of reasoning," explaining factors that influenced the choice.

These criteria summarize expert consensus opinion on how physicians can best assess medical decision-making capacity (Adams, 2000; Braddock, Edwards, Hasenberg, Laidley, & Levinson, 1999; Fellows, 1998; Larkin, Marco, & Abbott, 2001; Miller & Marin, 2000; Moskop, 1999; Thewes, FitzGerald, & Sulmasy, 1996). A patient's capacity to make medical decisions is not constant in every situation. Instead, patient capacity follows a "sliding scale" (Fellows, 1998). When a patient's choice involves the potential for significant harm (especially when this harm would be irreversible), the four criteria should be more stringently interpreted than when a patient selects a low-risk choice.

Capacity differs significantly from competence, although the terms are often interchanged. *Competence* is a legal designation regarding an individual's general ability to make autonomous decisions to protect his or her interests. Physicians cannot declare a patient incompetent; this requires a court hearing with expert testimony. Competence implies long-term ability to make most decisions, while a patient who lacks capacity to make medical decisions today may have capacity to do so tomorrow.

The opinion of another should be sought only when a patient is unable or unwilling to make his or her own decisions. The proxy or surrogate is asked to make a "substituted judgment," a choice based on an understanding of what the patient would want if he or she were able to speak for him- or herself. A patient can appoint an official *proxy* for health care decisions—a person the patient chooses explicitly when medically well who will speak for the patient should he or she later become unable to make decisions. As decision-making capacity waxes and wanes, so will the need for the proxy. A *surrogate* is a legal concept; a surrogate can only act on a patient's behalf after a court deems a patient incompetent and appoints a surrogate, or after court approval of a patient-selected surrogate. On rare occasions, in the absence of a proxy, the court may appoint a surrogate in an emergency where the patient is unable to speak for him- or herself. In either case, the physician must ensure that the proxy or surrogate has the capacity to make medical decisions and meets the four criteria outlined above.

In the case study, Dr. C must assess the decision-making capacity of both Mrs. E and Janice. If Mrs. E has capacity, it is her choice that counts, even if this creates a conflict with Janice. The point of balance between independence and safety may be in very different places for patients and their caregivers/families. A patient may be committed to his or her independence, even if the patient understands the risk of harm. The family may be more concerned about the patient's safety and more willing to give up the patient's independence. It may also be "easier" for family members if the patient is placed into some type of assisted living accommodation; there will be other caregivers available to help when needed. Conversely, patients may believe that they are a burden on caretakers and feel unworthy of expensive or time-intensive therapies, or they may fear that their caretakers will later criticize their choices. These underlying conflicts add complexity to decision-making in the ED.

For Mrs. E, the first questions are whether she can understand the diagnosis and comprehend the potential for benefit or harm from each treatment option. A physician can evaluate a patient's understanding by asking the patient to repeat the gist of the conversation, including the diagnosis and risks of each treatment presented. One study indicates that 40% of all elderly ED patients are cognitively impaired (Naughton, Moran, Kadah, Heman-Ackah, & Longano, 1995). Impaired individuals may lack medical decision-making capacity because they are not able to appreciate the consequences of their choices. No perfect test exists to differentiate these patients; intelligence scales, mental status exams, and dementia indexes do not predict a patient's medical decision-making capacity (Gerson, Counsell, Fontanarosa, & Smucker, 1994; McCusker, Bellavance, Cardin, Trepanier, Verdon, & Ardman, 1999). The ED physician and staff caring for the patient in the specific clinical situation must use clinical judgment to determine if the criteria for capacity are met (Mion, Palmer, Anetzberger, & Meldon, 2001).

In the case study, Mrs. E may be relying excessively on "normal" X rays, and because she does not experience much pain while lying flat, she may not fully grasp how her injury will impact her ability to live independently. On the other hand, her previous experience with a hospital admission suggests that she understands what "being admitted" means. Unfortunately, she also believes that "being admitted" to the acute care hospital will invariably lead to placement, against her wishes, in a nursing home, outcomes that are actually quite separate. Up to this point, the physician, social worker, and daughter have presented only two options to Mrs. E: admission versus returning home alone. It is important for the ED team to consider other potential options: short-term placement in a rehabilitation facility or staying at a family member's home with visiting nurse or aide assistance. Ensuring Mrs. E understands that an acute admission will not necessarily lead to nursing home placement and exploring alternatives to admission could help diffuse Mrs. E's anxiety.

The third criterion for capacity requires a choice to be reproducible over time. Mrs. E is not able to recall her medicine list or her daughter's phone number. Despite these memory deficiencies, her choice regarding admission remains stable over time. A patient with dementia may have short-term memory impairment while retaining the ability to weigh risks, benefits, and to make a choice based on personal beliefs and values. If this patient can demonstrate stability of choice by selecting the same desired option after repeated discussion regarding the situation and potential consequences of various options, that patient exhibits capacity even when he or she has severe memory deficits.

The final criterion for capacity is the patient's ability to explain factors influencing his or her choice. If this explanation is rational, even if the choice is contrary to medical recommendations, a patient is exhibiting capacity. Part of understanding the patient's reasoning is to ensure that the decision is voluntary. Early in Mrs. E's Emergency Department experience, it was clear that she opposed the idea of hospital admission. It would have been revealing then to determine what aspects of hospitalization were distasteful or worrisome to her, to see if these could be avoided during the proposed admission. For example, if Mrs. E associates hospitalization with surgery, pain, and prolonged postoperative recovery, her physician could reassure her that no surgery was anticipated. Instead, Mrs. E appears to disdain hospitalization because it entails a loss of her freedom and independence, and it would be deceitful to assure her that her fears were unfounded. Mrs. E articulates a chain of reasoning: her sisters have died in nursing homes, she does not feel sick, and even more difficult to ignore, she understands that her underlying disabilities are unlikely to improve after her injury heals, and thus she is unlikely to ever return to independent living.

What happens to Mrs. E? After further discussion and reassurance that she would retain her decision-making capacity as an inpatient, Mrs. E agreed to a short-term hospitalization to further assess her injuries and future living options.

CASE STUDY: NURSING HOME RESIDENT, EDGAR H.

Edgar H. is a 78-year-old man who has been residing in the Sunny Valley Elder facility for the last two years. He does not have much family in the area, though his granddaughter comes to visit him each month and was with him when he moved in. Despite having had a stroke, Edgar has been able to maintain some degree of communication with the staff. This morning, Sue, one of the nurse's aides, went to check on him as she does every weekday. She noticed that his eyes did not seem as bright as usual, and though he has never been a big talker, he did not respond with his usual couple of words, wink, or squeeze of the hand. This was Sue's first day back after the weekend, so she was not sure when the change developed, but she was concerned enough to tell her supervisor. The supervisor agreed that these conditions seemed a departure from Edgar's baseline, so an ambulance was called, and he was taken to the local hospital with a chief complaint of mental status changes. Edgar has always had a difficult time with hospitals, especially since the doctors and nurses always seem to either yell at him or ignore him when they are in his room. He is scared and unsure of what is going on around him and there are no familiar faces. When his wife was taken to the hospital two years ago for similar reasons, she did not make it back home.

The preceding scenario is not uncommon for patients who are transferred to EDs from nursing homes. There are often regular nursing home staff members who know the patient well enough to sense when something is awry. Frequently, the extent to which staff knows the patient has an impact on whether or not the patient is sent to an ED (Hutt, Ecord, Eilertsen, Frederickson, & Kramer, 2002). When various caregivers on different shifts take care of a patient, the exact time of onset of new symptoms is difficult to ascertain, made more difficult when the patient cannot communicate fully. Family members who do not visit frequently may be completely unaware of new developments. This leaves the receiving ED at the medical facility without an idea of the patient's baseline or where to begin an assessment for an "unresponsive patient" who has some degree of underlying dementia.

The ultimate goal for all parties involved (i.e., patient, family, nursing home staff, receiving facility staff) is obtaining the best and most appropriate care for the patient. Transitional care, as described by the American Geriatrics Society, consists of that which is necessary to ensure continuity of care as a patient moves from one care setting to another (Coleman & Boult, 2003). Again, communication is the key to achieving continuity. The groundwork for the communication should be laid before times of crisis or acute health changes because the chaos surrounding patient transfers does not allow for creating systems anew.

Fundamental information includes the reason why the patient was sent. In our scenario, Edgar cannot speak for himself and it would be dangerous for anyone in the ED to make assumptions about his true baseline. Who else knows him? Does his granddaughter know he is here? Is Sue still available to provide information on her understanding of his usual abilities and the changes in him? The following section deals with the perspective of each group involved and what each party could do to improve overall care for patients in Edgar's condition.

ESSENTIAL PATIENT INFORMATION

Nursing homes make an initial assessment when they receive a new client, but over time, the "baseline" mental status in a patient with dementia predictably declines. In the ED, an explicit explanation of both current "usual functioning" and the documented changes is important. Is what the ED staff sees of the patient's behavior and ability demonstrating someone who is acutely compromised or "back to baseline"? The answer can have vast implications for the speed and degree of emergency intervention (see Figure 6.2.). Current "usual" vital signs (temperature, heart rate, breathing rate, blood pressure, and oxygen levels) are important, because there is wide variability within the "normal" range. A patient could have "abnormal" numbers that would be dangerous to attempt to "correct" or normal values that actually represent acute changes for that patient.

Past medical problems can have a significant impact on ongoing health concerns. For that reason, a patient's thorough medical and surgical history should be part of any transfer. An appendectomy when a patient was seven years old can impact the evaluation for abdominal pain when he is seventy-seven. Additionally, current medications and allergies are of obvious importance since a single missed dose or accidental overdose of many medications can seriously impact health (Gurwitz, Field, Avorn, McCormick, Jain, & Eckler, et al., 2000).

The name and contact information of the patient's primary physician, next of kin, health care proxy, and durable power of attorney are also critical pieces for any receiving facility because these people know the patient best. Baseline function regarding activities of daily living like showering, brushing teeth, and dressing is important both for the ED and the inpatient setting. The ability to feed oneself and swallow and any history of aspiration should be included along with the patient's baseline communication skills, first language, and awareness of time and place (orientation).

"Noted this morning to be lethargic."

An extensive evaluation was performed in the ED including blood tests, CAT scans, urine tests, and Xrays. Nothing abnormal was found. When family arrived in the ED, it turned out the patient had been moved into a new room in the nursing home and was angry about it. He was at his baseline mental status.

"Fell, head laceration."

The patient could not explain what happened, and the nurse who had been there had left for the evening. Without any further information available, he was assumed to have fainted and struck his head while falling. He was placed into a cervical (neck) collar to prevent him from moving his neck, and a CAT scan of his head and the bones in his neck was performed. He became very agitated with lying flat while waiting for these tests and had to be sedated to hold still long enough for the scans to be performed. He had Xrays of his chest and abdomen, as well as blood tests. After the sedating medicine, he could not urinate, so a catheter had to be placed. The cut on his head was stitched. He spent over five hours in the ED. Because fainting in the elderly is most likely to be the result of an abnormal heart rhythm, he was admitted to the hospital although all of the other tests were negative or normal. Three days later he returned to the nursing home, where the nurse mentioned to the family that he had tripped and fallen against the wall (not to the ground) and the cut was from his glasses.

"Mrs. X (age 67) is usually continent but over the last two days has suddenly started needing a diaper. This morning, she is too weak to get out of bed and is much less verbal than her baseline."

Mrs. X had a urinary infection. She had a urine test and blood tests to check her electrolytes and kidney function. She returned to the nursing home and was much better in two days.

"Mr. P (age 72) caught his slipper on the leg of a chair and started to fall. He put his hand out to save himself and now his hand and wrist are swollen and painful. He was not unconscious before or after the fall and an aide saw him catch his foot but could not prevent him from falling. He normally says very little and his behavior after falling is normal."

Because the ED staff is sure the patient did not have syncope (fainting) as the cause of his fall, and that his mental status was normal for him, they were able to treat his broken wrist with a cast and return him to the nursing home. Without that specific information, he would likely have been admitted to the hospital for more testing and observation.

"Mrs. O (age 80) is usually quite active, chatting, and knitting. Over about the last three days, she has become much more lethargic, refusing to get out of bed and refusing to eat. She had not complained of pain anywhere and has not had any vomiting or diarrhea. She has had a little cough for the last few days."

Mrs. O was diagnosed with a large pneumonia. She received intravenous (IV) antibiotics but her breathing became more difficult. Her stated and written wishes were never to be placed on life support, so she was supported with care and medicines to keep her comfortable. She died on the third day in the hospital with her family around her.

FIGURE 6.2 Nursing home transfer note and outcome: the good, the bad, and the ugly.

All of the information just described, though onerous to assemble at time of transfer, is essential to quality care in an ED. Unfortunately, much of this information is lacking in many transfers from nursing homes to EDs or inpatient settings (Jones, Dwyer, White, & Firman, 1997). The time taken to clarify these issues early helps ensure better and more efficient medical care with less frustration for all involved. When such data are transferred with the patient, ED staff should recognize the benefit of the information and use it to optimize the patient's care.

Up to 40% of patients transferred to hospitals from nursing homes are admitted to the hospital (Ackermann, Kemle, Vogel, & Griffen, 1998). One study notes no significant differences in lengths of stay or outcomes in patients with similar conditions who were admitted directly to the hospital versus those who were admitted through the ED. Increased direct hospital admissions could decrease the amount of trauma for patients and families, while decreasing the number of opportunities for information to fall through the cracks (Aizen, Swartzman, & Clarfield, 2001).

All clients, within one week of initial admission to a skilled nursing home and every six months thereafter, should be engaged in a discussion regarding the extent of medical intervention they would want if they became direly ill and could not express their desires (Pauls, Singer, & Dubinsky, 2001). These conversations are often limited to whether patients would want to be intubated, have CPR, and be given medications to support blood pressure. But what about feeding tubes or dialysis? Would they want surgery? These conversations are essential and should occur prior to serious medical problems or presentation to an acute medical facility. Medical transfers made for acute health changes that seem minor can evolve rapidly into situations requiring heroic measures. Unfortunately, most patients transferred from skilled nursing facilities, and most of those who eventually have an indication for intubation, do not come with advanced directives specifying their desires (Lahn, Friedman, Bijur, Haughley, & Gallagher, 2001).

PATIENT AND FAMILY

A patient with baseline dementia may still have a very clear sense of when he or she feels well or ill, but be unable to communicate either. Edgar may have slept poorly the night prior to his interaction with the staff member because it was the second anniversary of his wife's death, but no one is aware of that fact aside from his granddaughter, who is not present. His anxiety level may heighten as he is told that he is going to the Emergency Department. He remembers that when his wife passed away, it was after a lengthy hospital course, with her last two weeks spent in the ICU. He remembers saying to himself that he would never want to have those kinds of measures for himself, but does not remember if he ever discussed this with his granddaughter or the staff at his nursing facility.

Edgar should be aware that while he has decision-making capacity, the medical care he receives is ultimately his choice. He needs to communicate his desires with those who care for him so that his wishes are respected. Edgar's granddaughter was unaware that he had been taken to the hospital. The ED called her while trying to elucidate his baseline and to what extent he would want extraordinary measures to resuscitate him. She told the staff that she remembered how distressing it was for Edgar to see his wife hooked up to machines and monitors in the ICU. She said he would want complete medical care, but if it came to machines and people pounding on his chest to keep him alive, he would rather be made comfortable and allowed to pass quietly.

In the end, Edgar did well. He was diagnosed with a small pneumonia and returned to the nursing home from the ED. Everyone involved was thankful that his issues were treatable. Edgar and his granddaughter were glad that they had thought about the tough issues earlier, but they also began to appreciate the need to clarify his wishes, so that if this happens again, they can focus on his health and well being.

CASE STUDY: RESUSCITATION, DOROTHY S.

Dorothy S. is a 79-year-old widow with a history of hypertension and emphysema who was diagnosed with Alzheimer's disease three years ago. Her dementia has been progressive, and more pronounced recently. Initially, she remained living in her home, making daily trips to a local senior center, with a homemaker to assist in cleaning and cooking. Her son paid her bills. One year ago, her family moved her to an assisted living facility where she lives in a two-room apartment and joins other residents for meals. A registered nurse administers Dorothy's medication on a routine basis. Over the last month, her family has become increasingly concerned about her apparent inattention to personal hygiene and the fact that she frequently does not recognize them when they visit. This week, she seemed to have a cold and a slight fever and was more confused on the telephone yesterday. Tonight, her niece found her on the floor next to her bed, quite disheveled, and with difficulty breathing. She was taken to a local ED and diagnosed with severe pneumonia. She is receiving 100% supplemental oxygen by a facemask and is on intravenous antibiotics and fluids. She is quite disoriented and keeps removing her oxygen mask. She seems fearful of the staff, although they constantly remind her that she is in the hospital and needs to cooperate with the therapy. The emergency physician approaches the family, Dorothy's son, daughter-in-law, and niece, to discuss the fact that Dorothy is not responding well to the current treatment, and to ask their wishes in the event that she is unable to breathe for herself or suffers a cardiac arrest. This has been a nagging worry for Dorothy's son, but he has not been willing to bring up these issues with his mother, his family, or his mother's primary care physician.

Decisions about how much intervention is desired by elderly demented patients are best made in the non-emergent situation. Individual patients and their families may have different beliefs and wishes for medical interventions. Those wishes must be discussed carefully and thoughtfully—optimally with the patient, any relevant family or other caregivers, and the patient's regular physician(s). When the patient has dementia, these conversations need to begin early—when the person is still able to clearly understand the issues involved and discuss his/her wishes. Medical resuscitation choices to be considered may include the use of artificial respiration (ventilators), medications to improve blood pressure, electrical shocks to the heart (defibrillation), and cardiopulmonary resuscitation (CPR). Less emergent options include whether technological means for delivering food and water (tube feedings), surgery, or hospital admission would be desired if needed. Some of these decisions may change over time as the dementia progresses; it may be useful to play "what if." Patients who are in good health and living at home may want "everything done" but be able to predict that their wishes for resuscitation would change if they became limited to living in a bed in a nursing home and could not speak or interact. These kinds of conversations can help families make good substituted judgments when patients are unable to speak for themselves.

Unfortunately, patients, families, and physicians often delay such complex and difficult conversations until the emergent situation occurs. Urgent decisions may have to be made without the full participation of the ill patient. Several issues impact the resuscitation of the ill elderly at the end-of-life in the emergency department. Caregiver, proxy, and family reactions to what may be an acute terminal illness may make it hard for them to make a unified decision in an emergent situation. If information on individual choices is not readily available to the emergency physician, potentially unwanted and invasive therapy may be initiated in the ED when patients become unstable and at risk of imminent death. To make good treatment choices, elderly patients, their families, caregivers, and physicians need to be aware of the potential outcomes of resuscitation in elderly demented patients, and understand the use of advance directives.

Medical outcomes of elderly patients have been studied in the cases of both acute hospitalization and cardiopulmonary arrest. Elderly patients with end-stage dementia have poorer outcomes compared to those without cognitive impairments following hospitalization for hip fracture or pneumonia (Morrison & Siu, 2000). In a prospective study of 235 patients 70 years or older who were admitted to an acute care hospital over two years with these diagnoses, the six-month mortality for elderly patients with end-stage dementia was much higher than for patients who were cognitively intact. Six-month mortality for severely demented patients with pneumonia was 53%, as compared to 13% for intact patients. Similarly, six-month mortality for severely demented patients with hip fracture was 55%, as compared to 12% for intact patients. In addition, elderly patients who are hospitalized are less likely to recover baseline activities of daily living and more likely to develop new functional deficits during hospitalization (Covinsky, Counsell, Palmer, Fortinsky, Stewart, & Kresevic, et al., 2003). In addition, there is a significant interaction between age and baseline functional status as these factors impact mortality. Mayer-Oakes found that patients older than 75 years with functional limitations (no longer able to live alone or take full care of themselves) were almost six times more likely to die in a hospital following medical intensive care (a stay in the ICU or intensive care unit). (Mayer-Oakes, Oye, & Leake, 1991)

Outcomes for cardiopulmonary resuscitation (CPR) in elderly patients are poor. Of 503 patients over the age of 70 who received CPR, only 3.8% survived to hospital discharge. (Murphy, Murray, Robinson, & Campion, 1989) Elderly patients whose pulse stopped outside of the hospital and those whose hearts were not fibrillating (with asystole or electromechanical dissociation) had uniformly dismal outcomes. Elderly patients whose hearts stop in-hospital and survive resuscitation are at significantly increased risk of functional deterioration post-resuscitation, are often profoundly disabled after CPR, and are less likely to survive to hospital discharge. (FitzGerald et al., 1997)

For all of these reasons, potential medical outcomes in elderly demented patients who require acute hospitalization or are at risk for cardiopulmonary arrest should be discussed with the patients and their families and should be understood by treating physicians. The risks and benefits of treatment options can be weighed by the patients and/or proxies, based on the patients' stated goals at the time they were competent. Based on these goals, a range of care, from resuscitation to comfort and palliation, can be decided upon. If patients' goals for care are continuously reassessed when events such as hospitalization or loss of activities of daily living occur, advance medical planning can proceed accordingly.

ADVANCE DIRECTIVES

Advance directives are proactive, written forms that indicate what a patient's choices would have been for medical treatment if he or she had decision-making capacity at the time decisions must be made (Sanders, 1999). Advance directives attempt to extend and preserve a patient's autonomy over medical decision-making in the event of temporary or permanent mental incapacity. Advance directives consist of living wills, durable powers of attorney (identifying a health care proxy), and limited "do not attempt resuscitation" forms. Living wills express the patient's wishes in the event of acute or end-of-life illness if the patient's mental status has deteriorated such that he or she is unable to assert decision-making capacity. The directives may outline a patient's specific wishes for various therapeutic interventions as well as indicate that a patient chooses death over continued therapy and prolonged life. A durable power of attorney is a written document that assigns a chosen surrogate to make health care decisions for the patient in the event of mental incapacity. The most common hierarchy of surrogate decision makers is spouse, adult children, and siblings. "Do not attempt resuscitation" (DNR) forms provide written instructions in the event of cardiopulmonary arrest.

The Patient Self-Determination Act of 1991 (42 U.S.C. §§ 1395 ccm 1396a, 1994) was passed by Congress with the intention of enhancing an individual's control of his or her medical treatment by extending and protecting the patient's autonomy when he or she becomes incapable of expressing wishes for care. The Act mandates that all health care institutions that receive Medicare and Medicaid funding must advise and educate patients about advance directives. Since implementation of the Patient Self-Determination Act, an increased prevalence of advance directive documentation in nursing home medical records has been reported in some studies (Bradley, Wetle, & Horwitz, 1998). Fried and Gillick (1994) reported that 40% of geriatric patients chose some limitation of diagnostic testing or treatment in the six months prior to their death. During their final illnesses, 89% of geriatric patients had some limitations of treatment, primarily CPR and intubation (mechanical ventilation).

Despite these studies, only a minority of elderly persons completes advance directives. Of 401 critically ill elderly patients in an ICU setting, only 5% had prior advance directives (Goodman, Tarnoff, & Slotman, 1998). Hispanic and African-American patients are even less likely to complete these health care documents (Morrison, Zayas, Mulvihill, Baskin, & Meier., 1998). Even when advance directives have been completed, they may not be transmitted to the hospital with the patient (Jones, Dwyer, White, & Firman, 1997).

If advance directives are transmitted to treating providers, care may still not be consistent with the patient's stated wishes. For example, Danis and colleagues (1991) studied outcome events for 126 nursing home residents with documented advance directives. The investigators prospectively followed these patients over a two-year period to determine how end-of-life care compared with advance directive preferences. They found that medical treatment was inconsistent with the patient's written wishes in 25% of outcome events. Unwanted aggressive treatment included mechanical ventilation, surgery, CPR, and tube feeding. In an ICU setting, the presence of an advance directive was not associated with any difference in the quantity and level of care received by these patients, as compared to matched patients without advance directives (Goodman, Tarnoff, & Slotman, 1998).

The predictions of primary care physicians and health care proxies about a patient's wishes have not been shown to be accurate. In response to hypothetical scenarios requiring cardiopulmonary resuscitation, patients predicted that their physicians and family members would accurately represent their wishes. However, neither physicians nor family members were able to predict the patient's wishes for resuscitation in the setting of diminished mental capacity (Seckler, Meier, Mulvihill, Cammer Paris, 1991). In a more recent study of physicians' discussions of advance directive planning with patients, physicians were more accurately able to identify the patient's surrogate, but there was poor agreement between physicians and their patients regarding treatment preferences in 18 of 20 resuscitation scenarios (Gischer, Tulsky, Rose, Siminoff, & Arnold, 1998).

All of these factors impact the emergency treatment and resuscitation of elderly, demented patients who are vulnerable to potentially invasive, painful procedures and unwanted resuscitation in the ED. Continuous, ongoing assessment and discussion of a patient's goals and desires for care at the end–of-life are necessary to establish understanding among patient, family, surrogate, and primary care physician. These goals should be understood in light of the potential outcomes of acute illness or cardiopulmonary arrest, and advance-planning decisions should be made accordingly. Advance directives should also be continuously reassessed and the information readily available and transferable in the event of emergent transport to the hospital. Clearly written statements of the patient's desires can help optimize care in the ED and should be routinely included in the medical information transferred with the patient. Through continuing reevaluation and discussion, a patient can ensure that his or her personal medical autonomy and dignity be maintained if diminished mental capacity or progressive dementia is complicated by acute, life-threatening illness.

In Dorothy's case, no one knew her wishes. She was intubated and placed on mechanical ventilation. She was admitted to the ICU from the ED and underwent the placement of a central line, urinary catheter, and arterial line. Initially, her oxygenation improved, but over the course of the next several days, she got worse. A lung collapsed and a chest tube had to be inserted to re-inflate it. She required multiple medicines to support her blood pressure, and more to keep her sedated to tolerate everything that was going on. Finally, her kidneys shut down, and at a meeting between family members and the treating physicians and nurses, the decision was made not to start dialysis. The group agreed to stop all life support, and she died within a few hours.

CONCLUSIONS AND RECOMMENDATIONS

It is a fact of life that people become unexpectedly sick or injured and need emergency care. Patients with dementia have particular difficulty negotiating the process of care in the Emergency Department and present special complexities to their health care providers. Families, caregivers, and physicians can do several things to assist *before* the emergency happens. Keeping careful track of patients' current levels of functioning, along with their medical histories, medications, allergies, and long-term wishes in written form helps physicians and nurses optimize care in the ED. Documented details like the fact that a patient only hears out of the left ear and often lip reads but needs glasses on to do so make it much easier for the ED providers to ensure that the patient gets what he or she needs.

As noted, Figure 6.1 shows a type of form used to facilitate information transfer. It spells out exactly the person's current level of functioning and specific medical problems and identifies the appropriate people to contact for more information (the health care proxy and the primary physician), and it contains information about the patient's wishes. For example, if a patient enters the ED and is unable to speak in sentences and cannot undress him- or herself, the ED team would recognize that the patient needed a careful evaluation to identify the problem. For another patient with more severe dementia, knowing that he or she is unable to speak in sentences or get undressed without help at baseline would mean less testing. A similar form could be used whether the person is living at home or in an assisted living, rehabilitation, or nursing facility.

Circumstances change as time progresses. Unfortunately, in dementia, there is a progressive loss of abilities. Therefore, every few months, information on the form should be updated. Using such a tool stimulates the proactive reassessment of living choices, treatment preferences, and resuscitation plans. The information needs to be shared with all relevant caregivers and any treating physicians. In particular, resuscitation discussions should begin when the person can still participate in the discussion.

In addition to making sure that ED providers know as much as possible about the patient, having a familiar family member or caregiver stay with the patient is an important part of improving the demented patient's stay in the ED. A familiar face can help calm the patient when the wait seems long or there are many distractions and unfamiliar people.

At the same time, ED staff can work to ensure that patients with dementia are exposed to as little chaos as possible in the ED. Dementia patients can be placed in a quieter area. When dealing with dementia patients, calm, clear, one-step instructions from one person at a time help prevent confusion. Being proactive about meals and regular medicine can fend off escalations of extreme behavior or inappropriate attempts to leave. Ensuring that patients are comfortable by offering pillows or extra blankets is helpful. Optimal interactions may depend on the patients' use of hearing aids or glasses. Finally, providers need to be attentive to patients' needs for pain medicine.

Effective communication from patients, families, caregivers, and nursing home staff to the ED providers is the key to optimizing the ED care of demented patients. When information about current levels of functioning, medical problems, medications, and desires for resuscitation are available, patients are more likely to get efficient, effective care. At the same time, ED providers must understand the progressive nature of dementia and be able to cope effectively with patients at each stage of the disease.

REFERENCES

Ackermann, R. J., Kemle, K. A., Vogel, R. L., & Griffin, R. C., Jr. (1998). Emergency department use by nursing home residents. *Annals of Emergency Medicine, 31*(6), 749–757.

Adams, J. (2000). *Assessing the decision-making capacity of an emergency patient.* ACEP Scientific Assembly, Philadelphia.

Aizen, E., Swartzman, R., & Clarfield, A. M. (2001). Hospitalization of nursing home residents in an acute-care geriatric department: Direct versus emergency room admission. *Israel Medical Association Journal, 3*(10), 734–738.

Birrer, R., Singh, U., & Kumar, D. N. (1999). Disability and dementia in the emergency department. *Emergency Medicine Clinics of North America, 17*(2), 505–517, xiii.

Braddock, C. H., III, Edwards, K. A., Hasenberg, N. M., Laidley, T. L., & Levinson, W. (1999). Informed decision-making in outpatient practice: Time to get back to basics. *Journal of the American Medical Association, 282*(24), 2313–2320.

Bradley, E. H., Wetle, T., & Horwitz, S. M. (1998). The Patient Self-Determination Act and advance directive completion in nursing homes. *Archives of Family Medicine, 7,* 417–423.

Coleman, E. A., & Boult, C. (2003). The American Geriatrics Society Health Care Systems Committee. Improving the quality of transitional care for persons with complex care needs. *Journal of the American Geriatrics Society, 51,* 556–557.

Covinsky, K. E., Palmer, R. M., Fortinsky, R. H., Counsell, S. R., Stewart, A. L., & Kresevic, D., et al. (2003). Loss of independence in activities of daily living in older adults hospitalized with medical illnesses: Increased vulnerability with age. *Journal of the American Geriatrics Society, 51,* 451–458.

Danis, M., Southerland, L. I., Garrett, J. M., Smith, J. L., Hielema, F., & Pickard, C. G., et al. (1991). A prospective study of advance directives for life-sustaining care. *New England Journal of Medicine, 324,* 882–888.

Eriksson, S. (1999). Social and environmental contributants to delirium in the elderly. *Dementia and Geriatric Cognitive Disorders, 10*(5), 350–352.

Ettinger, W. H., Casani, J. A., Coon, P. J. , Muller, D. C., Piazza-Appel, K. (1987). Patterns of use of the emergency department by elderly patients. *Journal of Gerontology, 42*(6), 638–642.

Feldt, K. S., Ryden, M. B., & Miles, S. (1998). Treatment of pain in cognitively impaired compared with cognitively intact older patients with hip-fracture. *Journal of the American Geriatric Society, 46*(9), 1079–1085.

Fellows, L. K. (1998). Competency and consent in dementia. *Journal of the American Geriatrics Society, 46*(7), 922–926.

FitzGerald, J. D., Wenger, N. S., Califf, R. M., Phillips, R. S., Desbiens, N. A., & Liu, H., et al. (1997). Functional status among survivors of in-hospital cardiopulmonary resuscitation. *Archives of Internal Medicine, 157,* 72–76.

Fried, T. R., & Gillick, M. R. (1994). Medical decision-making in the last six months of life: choices about limitation of care. *Journal of the American Geriatrics Society, 42,* 303–307.

Gerson, L. W., Counsell, S. R., Fontanarosa P. B., & Smucker W. D. (1994). Case finding for cognitive impairment in elderly emergency department patients. *Annals of Emergency Medicine, 23*(4), 813–817.

Gischer, G. S., Tulsky, J. A., Rose, M. R., Siminoff, L. A, & Arnold, R. M. (1998). Patient knowledge and physician predictions of treatment preferences after discussion of advance directives. *Journal of General Internal Medicine, 13,* 447–454.

Goodman, M. D., Tarnoff, M., & Slotman, G. J. (1998). Effect of advance directives on the management of elderly critically ill patients. *Critical Care Medicine, 26,* 701–704.

Gurwitz, J. H., Field, T. S., Avorn, J., McCormick, D., Jain, S., & Eckler, M., et al. (2000). Incidence and preventability of adverse drug events in nursing homes. *American Journal of Medicine, 109,* 87–94.

Hustey, F. M., Meldon, S., & Palmer, R. (2000). Prevalence and documentation of impaired mental status in elderly emergency department patients. *Academic Emergency Medicine, 7*(10), 1166.

Hutt, E., Ecord, M., Eilertsen, T. B., Frederickson, E., & Kramer, A. M. (2002). Precipitants of emergency room visits and acute hospitalization in short-stay Medicare nursing home residents. *Journal of the American Geriatrics Society, 50*(2), 223–229.

Jones, J. S., Dwyer, P. R., White, L. J., & Firman, R. (1997). Patient transfer from nursing home to emergency department: Outcomes and policy implications. *Academic Emergency Medicine, 4*(9), 908–915.

Lahn, M., Friedman, B., Bijur, P., Haughey, M., & Gallagher, E. J. (2001). Advance directives in skilled nursing facility residents transferred to emergency departments. *Academic Emergency Medicine, 8*(12), 1158–1162.

Lambe, S., Washington, D. L., Fink, A., Laouri, M., Liu, H., & Scura Fosse, J., et al. (2002). Waiting times in California's emergency departments. *Annals of Emergency Medicine, 41*(1), 35–44.

Lammers, R. L., Roiger, M., Rice, L., Overton, D. T., & Cucos, D. (2003). The effect of a new emergency medicine residency program on patient length of stay in a community hospital emergency department. *Academic Emergency Medicine, 10*(7), 725–730.

Larkin, G. L., Marco, C. A., & Abbott, J. T. (2001). Emergency determination of decision-making capacity: Balancing autonomy and beneficence in the emergency department. *Academic Emergency Medicine, 8*(3), 282–284.

Lewis, L. M., Miller, D. K., Morley, J. E. (1995). Unrecognized delirium in ED geriatric patients. *American Journal of Emergency Medicine, 13*(2), 142–145.

Mayer-Oakes, S. A., Oye, R. K., & Leake, B. (1991). Predictors of mortality in older patients following medical intensive care: The importance of functional status. *Journal of the American Geriatrics Society, 39,* 862–868.

McCusker, J., Bellavance, F., Cardin, S., Trepanier, S., Verdon, J., & Ardman, O. (1999). Detection of older people at increased risk of adverse health outcomes after an emergency visit: The ISAR screening tool. *Journal of the American Geriatrics Society, 47*(10), 1229–1237.

Miller, S. S., & Marin, D. B. (2000). Assessing capacity. *Emergency Medicine Clinics of North America, 18*(2), 233–242, viii.

Mion, L. C., Palmer, R. M., Anetzberger, G. L. & Meldon, S. W. (2001). Establishing a case-finding and referral system for at-risk older individuals in the emergency department setting: The SIGNET model. *Journal of the American Geriatrics Society, 49*(10), 1379–1386.

Morrison, R. S., Zayas, L. H., Mulvihill, M., Baskin, S. A., & Meier, D. E. (1998). Barriers to completion of health care proxies. An examination of ethnic differences. *Archives of Internal Medicine, 158,* 2493–2497.

Morrison, R. S., & Siu, A. L. (2000). Survival in end-stage dementia following acute illness. *Jornal of the American Medical Association 284,* 47–52.

Moskop, J. C. (1999). Informed consent in the emergency department. *Emergency Medicine Clinics of North America*, 17(2), 327–340, ix-x.

Murphy, D. J, Murray, A. M., Robinson, B. E., & Campion, E. W. (1989). Outcomes of cardiopulmonary resuscitation in the elderly. *Annals of Internal Medicine*, 111, 199–205.

Naughton, B. J., Moran, M. B., Kadah, H., Heman-Ackah, Y., & Longano, J. (1995). Delirium and other cognitive impairment in older adults in an emergency department. *Annals of Emergency Medicine*, 25(6), 751–755.

Partovi, S. N., Nelson, B. K., Bryan, E. D., & Walsh, M. J. (2001). Faculty triage shortens emergency department length of stay. *Academic Emergency Medicine*, 8, 990–995.

Pauls, M. A., Singer, P. A., & Dubinsky, I. (2001). Communicating advance directives from long-term care facilities to emergency departments. *Journal of Emergency Medicine*, 21(1), 83–89.

Sanders, A. B. (1999). Advance directives. *Emergency Medicine Clinics of North America*, 17, 519–526.

Seckler, A. B., Meier, D. E., Mulvihill, M., & Cammer Paris, B. E. (1991). Substituted judgment: How accurate are proxy predictions? *Annals of Internal Medicine*, 115, 92–98.

Shah, M. N., Rathouz, P. J., & Chin (2001). Emergency department utilization by noninstitutionalized elders. *Academy of Emergency Medicine*, 8(3), 267–273.

Sugarman, J., McCrory, D. C., Hubal, R. C. (1998). Getting meaningful informed consent from older adults: A structured literature review of empirical research. *Journal of the American Geriatrics Society*, 46(4), 517–524.

The Patient Self-Determination Act 42 U.S.C. §§ 1395 ccm 1396a (1994).

Thewes, J., FitzGerald, D., Sulmasy, D. P. (1996). Informed consent in emergency medicine: Ethics under fire. *Emergency Medicine Clinics of North America*, 14(1), 245–254.

The Inpatient Experience from the Perspective of the Isolated Adult with Alzheimer's Disease

Charles E. Drebing and Tamara Harden

Ten to twenty percent of adults with Alzheimer's disease (AD) who are living in the community are living alone and have no identifiable caregiver or person in charge of overseeing their care. These isolated elders often underutilize outpatient care and present particular challenges for providers in hospital settings. The impact of isolation is particularly critical in the process of admission to inpatient care, the collection of accurate clinical data, compliance with treatment, and discharge planning. Strategies for working with this isolated group within a hospital setting are discussed, including strategies for addressing entry into care, communication between professional and nonprofessional caregivers, clinical data collection, and addressing the lack of informal support. Several case studies illustrate the potential roles hospitalization can play in the course of dementia care.

CASE STUDY: MS. WATKINS

When Ms. Watkins heard that her closest friend was dying of cancer, she felt she should move out of her apartment and move in with her friend on the other side of town, so that she could oversee her care and keep her safe. When her friend died two years later, Ms. Watkins was still living in her apartment. The first symptoms of her dementia became apparent to the building staff a year later, though she showed no awareness herself. Ms. Watkins began to complain that she could not find her belongings and suggested that her neighbors may be stealing from her. When staff would suggest that this was impossible because of her locked door, she became belligerent. She was increasingly embroiled in arguments with staff and fellow elderly housing residents, leaving her with the reputation of a troublemaker. Staff members were aware that she probably had dementia, but they were more aware that she caused them a great deal of work in trying to keep the peace. They were also increasingly concerned about her ability to live safely in the building. While she had home-delivered meals, she was leaving the food in her home until it was moldy. Her apartment was cluttered with paper, and there was concern that she might start a fire with her stove.

In addition to her behavioral problems, she had high blood pressure, which often went uncontrolled because she forgot to take her medication. One day she passed out, fell, and was admitted to a hospital emergency room. Her blood pressure was brought under control after she was given her medicine. During their attempt to gather her history, the hospital staff noted that she was clearly a poor historian and appeared very confused. Not being clear regarding the nature of her confusion, she was admitted for a more thorough work-up. Efforts to complete the evaluation were hampered by difficulty getting a complete history from anyone. Ms. Watkins could not answer the clinician's questions, and she had no family that she could identify who could provide information. The staff at her elder housing apartment provided some background, but they knew little about her medical history. Her physician was contacted, and he was able to talk about her history of high blood pressure, but he was not aware of her memory complaints.

Despite the limited history, the hospital staff quickly concluded that Ms. Watkins suffered from probable Alzheimer's disease (AD) and that, given her current living situation and the lack of any family to take her in, she needed placement into a long-term care facility. What they did not anticipate was the challenge in discharging her. Adults with dementia require special long-term care facilities. Ms. Watkins was less demented than many residents of special Alzheimer's programs, most of whom were cared for at home by family until a later stage of the illness, when families simply could not manage them anymore. Placing a higher functioning adult with early-stage dementia and clear behavioral problems is often a challenge.

Unfortunately for Ms. Watkins, her discharge planning faced a more serious challenge. After further data collection, hospital staff found that Ms. Watkins was not an American citizen. She had moved to the United States from Europe twenty years ago. Funding therefore became a major hurdle, one that the staff was unable to overcome. Ms. Watkins had depleted all of her funds years ago, during an earlier illness. She was not eligible for Medicare or Medicaid because of her citizenship. The staff considered returning her to her prior home, but the staff at the elderly housing, relieved to have Ms. Watkins out of their building, had quickly moved another resident into her apartment. While the hospital staff looked for a creative solution, Ms. Watkins settled into the geriatrics unit. She had no real need to be there; her medical problems were easily managed. Her behavioral symptoms were now well managed also, and so she was comfortable and compliant. By her 31st day on the ward, the hospital staff was desperately trying to find some place for her to go, as they watched the cost of her care rise every day with no end in sight.

This case represents some of the potential problems hospitals face in working with a relatively unstudied group of Alzheimer's patients—those who live alone and have no family caregivers coordinating their care. The incidences of both living alone and dementia increase with age (Webber, Fox, & Burnette, 1994). Currently, over four million people in the United States are afflicted with AD, and this number is expected to reach 13.2 million in 2050 (Alzheimer's Association, 2003; Drebing, 1999; Grossberg, 2003). Most people with AD live in the community, and many are living alone. Fortunately, many of those living alone are receiving care and supervision from family (Drebing, 1999). This group has been getting more attention recently, as professionals seek to find ways to help their families support them (Newhouse, Niebuhr, Stroud, & Newhouse, 2001). Unfortunately, there is a more vulnerable subgroup of those living alone: those who have no significant involvement of family or friends. There is little research data available for this group. While an average of 100 empirical studies are published each year examining family caregivers and caregiving of persons with AD, it is difficult to find studies focusing on persons with AD who do not have family caregivers. One of the reasons is clear: It is much more difficult for researchers to collect data about this group. Who will provide the information for the isolated adult with AD? The resulting gap in our knowledge represents an important limitation in our ability to address the clinical needs of this particularly vulnerable group. This chapter presents a review of what is known about isolated elders living with dementia, a discussion of the challenges these adults represent for hospital settings, and strategies for clinicians working in inpatient settings to address these challenges.

THE IMPACT OF ISOLATION ON ILLNESSES AND CARE

In general, social isolation in older adults has a number of undesirable correlates, including lower income, poorer physical health, poorer functional status, and higher mortality (Leveist, Sellers, Brown, & Nickerson, 1998). The exact role that isolation plays in health outcomes in general remains unclear. While some have suggested that it is merely a correlate of declining health, the available data suggest a more complex role (Leveist et al., 1998; Rathbone & Hashimi, 1982). Social isolation appears to have a significant relationship to health outcomes independent of physical health and appears to play a moderating role in outcome, either through health-promoting behaviors or through its relationship to socioenvironmental and psychological factors such as depression (Leveist et al., 1998; Rathbone & Hashimi, 1982; Tuokko, MacCourt, & Heath, 1999). When it comes to health care utilization, isolated elders are at risk for underutilization of needed services, particularly outpatient services (Ebly, Hogan, & Rockwood, 1999).

Participating in health care is, in one sense, a part of social behavior. People talk about going to the doctor; they tell each other to go for care; and they help each other get to providers. It is predictable that those who are socially isolated will be less involved in outpatient care. The inverse is true of the relationship between isolation and institutional care. Isolation is associated with an increase in the risk of institutionalization independent of self-reported health status (U.S. Department of Health and Human Services, 1988). Those without the social resources to support them safely in the community are placed into settings where professional supports substitute for family and friends (Steinback, 1992).

Isolation and Dementia

While the role family caregivers play in the care of adults with AD has received a great deal of research attention, the impact of having no family caregiver coordinating or providing care has been relatively unstudied. Early studies of caregiving suggested that virtually all adults with dementia live with family caregivers or in residential care settings. Subsequent epidemiological studies showed this assumption to be unfounded. In the Epidemiological Catchment Area Survey, 24% of adults with severe cognitive impairment were living alone, with up to 44% in urban areas living alone (U.S. Department of Health and Human Services, 1988).

Across the six California Alzheimer Disease Diagnostic and Treatment Centers, 21% of subjects with Alzheimer's disease and related disorders (ADRD) were living alone (Fox, Lindeman, & Benjamin, 1988). Of those living alone, approximately 50%, or 10 to 22% of the total samples, reportedly did not have an identifiable friend or family member providing significant care or oversight. Based on these figures, a conservative estimate of 10% or between 400,000 and 800,000 Americans with AD likely live alone and have no easily identifiable family caregiver, with those living in urban areas being twice as likely to be isolated (Fox et al., 1988; U.S. Department of Health and Human Services, 1988; Newhouse et al., 2001).

The few studies that have looked at people living alone with dementia have found that living alone is a barrier to proper diagnosis, treatment, and appropriately timed institutionalization (Webber et al., 1994). The research has also shown that elders living alone with dementia are particularly at risk for adverse outcomes such as unmet needs, self-neglect, and injury, which can lead to early institutionalization (Minkler, 1986; Rathbone & Hashimi, 1982). In adults with dementia, isolation has been associated with a lower probability of initiating treatment and a lower likelihood of using outpatient services relative to their nonisolated counterparts (Raschko, 1991). Instead, they appear to have a higher risk of being hospitalized early in the course of their illness (Webber et al., 1994), suggesting that formal care often substitutes for informal care, with a resulting increase in cost and a drop in the compatibility between need and level of care.

The following study focuses on elders with dementia living alone without identifiable caregivers coordinating their care.

OVERVIEW OF THE VULNERABLE ISOLATED PERSONS PROJECT

Funded in 2000 by the Alzheimer's Association, the Vulnerable Isolated Persons Project (VIP) is a research study of isolated adults with Alzheimer's disease. This three-year project was conducted in the metro-Boston area through a partnership among the Bedford VA Medical Center, the Boston University School of Medicine, and the Alzheimer's Association Massachusetts Chapter. One hundred twenty-eight isolated older adults were referred to the project from a range of sources, including social service, medical providers, and neighbors or family of isolated seniors. Slightly over a third were excluded due to an unwillingness to participate by either the patient or the patient's family member. Another third were excluded because they did not meet the study criteria either for isolation or AD. The remaining forty isolated older adults with possible/probable AD signed consent to participate in the project. Sixty percent of this sample was female, and the average age of the group was 81.5 years. Half of the sample was Caucasian and 40% was African-American. More than half had never been married, and the mean number of children was 1.2. Given the challenge of finding valid data from this group, we collected data from at least five of the following sources: the isolated adult, his or her medical provider, his or her medical record, his or her social service provider, a family member, and a friend or neighbor. Conclusions about the current state of patient health, the current number and types of services received, and currently unmet needs were developed by consensus after reviewing all available data.

While all VIP project participants were evaluated and diagnosed with possible or probable AD, prior to entry only 29% had been formally diagnosed with AD and only 65% had memory impairment or other cognitive symptoms noted in their medical records. Despite meeting criteria for isolation, most were still receiving some form of informal care, typically from neighbors or family. Most were seeing their physicians on a regular basis, with an average of three visits in the year prior to admission to the study. Only 29% had been diagnosed with AD and only 12% had been diagnosed with dementia or had any mention of cognitive symptoms of dementia in their medical records. Most were found to have been hospitalized or evaluated in a hospital setting within the course of their dementia. The role of the hospital contact fell into a few common patterns. Ms. Watkins represents a small group for whom hospitalization was a particularly costly or ineffective method of care. Based on our experience, we have drawn a number of conclusions.

Challenges That Isolated Elders with Dementia Pose to Hospital Staff

Patients are supposed to be active participants in their own care. Being an effective patient, that is, playing the patient role in a way that contributes toward a positive outcome of care, requires both effort and ability on the patient's part. The effective patient must initiate treatment, make suitable arrangements to ensure that appropriate treatment takes place, attend appointments as needed, present needed information to the provider, listen and understand the provider's information and feedback, make decisions about his or her care based on that feedback, and then follow through with recommendations and treatments initiated by the provider. In hospital settings, the patient role may be more passive because of the available structure, which can ensure availability for services. At the same time, hospital settings can demand more of the patient than other settings. There are more providers and staff making varied demands on the patient—demands for information, compliance, and follow-up. In particular, listening and digesting information provided by clinicians, making decisions about care, and following through with treatment and discharge recommendations are more daunting when there are more people providing the information and the recommendations.

When a patient's ability to play his or her part effectively is compromised by AD, in most cases it falls to the family to be the facilitator of health care. In the absence of family or another informal caregiver, it is unclear what happens.

Initiation of treatment: First, patients appear to be less likely to initiate discussions with their providers about their dementia symptoms, often leaving the providers in the dark about the problem until the symptoms are pronounced. Of the forty participants in the VIP study, less than a third had a diagnosis of AD or dementia in the medical chart, and almost half had no mention of any dementia symptom of any type. Isolated adults are less likely to be initiating conversations with their providers about other medical problems as well, resulting in undiagnosed and untreated medical conditions as demonstrated by the case of Ms Watkins.

Admission to inpatient care. Admission to the hospital can result in both predictable and unpredictable problems for adults with dementia. The move to an unfamiliar setting and routine can increase their confusion and agitation, making their dementia more apparent and more disabling. One of the key roles family caregivers play is in helping the patient understand and adapt to changes. Family members have typically learned the best ways to communicate with and to soothe their relatives with AD. They also help providers understand the patients' symptoms and reactions, and they can be helpful in teaching providers how to work with patients to minimize resistance. For isolated adults, there is often no one playing this role; no one to calm and soothe the agitated patient; no one to help the patient find some understanding of his or her new environment. No one is there to reframe the situation for the providers so that they see the person and the larger picture. While staff is well experienced and often very talented at discovering some of this information, the isolated adult with dementia represents, at minimum, an additional behavior management challenge for even the most dedicated providers. Given the time demands of inpatient care, pharmacological measures to manage the confused patient may be more common among isolated patients than for those with family caregivers.

Providing an accurate history: Ms. Watkins had failed to give her physician accurate data about her blood pressure, probably because she did not remember to tell him or possibly she failed to recognize what she was experiencing. When she was seen in the emergency room, the staff noticed evidence of her dementia, but they had no available history of the symptoms, as Ms. Watkins could provide little if any personal or medical history. As is common with providers for these isolated adults, the hospital staff had a clinical history that had major gaps, which made it difficult to diagnose and treat new conditions and to monitor progress with existing conditions.

Complying with treatment: Not surprisingly, we found that many VIP participants were not complying with medical treatments initiated by their providers. One participant showed us a drawer full of empty prescription medication containers that had been filled two days before. He had no memory about what happened to the medicine and would have gone without medication without our intervention. Another had been advised by his hospital clinicians upon discharge to use a moisturizer on the psoriasis on his legs. In the patient's compromised mind, that recommendation evolved over several days into the recommendation that he put kerosene on his legs, which he began doing regularly because he believed his doctors told him to do so.

The case of Ms. Watkins demonstrates how the difficulty with treatment compliance can lead to hospitalization of isolated adults with dementia. We also met many physicians who were refusing to write prescriptions for VIP participants because they were aware of the potential for noncompliance and dangerous misuse of prescription medications. Unfortunately, lack of needed medications represents a real risk as well.

Discharge planning: For those hospital clinicians who do acknowledge and address dementia in isolated adults, discharge planning can be a challenge. As noted earlier, this isolated group is at risk for earlier institutionalization, probably because of concerns about safety and the lack of family supports for outpatient treatment. Like Ms. Watkins, they are typically higher functioning than adults with dementia who have sufficient family supports to live in the community until their dementia increases severely, and so do not fit well in special dementia care units. If placed in such a unit, they often have sufficient insight to realize where they are and what is going on around them, leading to emotional distress and to management challenges for the program staff. Recognizing the potential decline faced by adults with dementia, staff involved in discharge planning may feel that discharge back home is the best disposition for the patient. Arranging for enough adjunct services to support treatment and safety becomes a larger task, because a full range of needs must be addressed.

Addressing patient safety issues following discharge is a critical element of discharge planning. Collecting information about safety risks and potentially dangerous incidents such as fires, falls, and medication errors in this population confirmed for us that these isolated adults with dementia do present elevated risks for a range of safety hazards. Providers who look closely enough to see the reality of these patients' daily lives are likely be to be concerned about how to keep them safe. To avoid responsibility for accidents or for finding ways to avoid them, some providers choose not to delve too deeply into cases of isolated adults with AD. In another version of "don't ask, don't tell," providers may find it safer not to find out about functional deficits. They conclude that, short of institutionalization, there is little that can be done to keep these patients safe. Such conclusions may explain how half of the cases in our study had no documented evidence of dementia in their medical records.

The case of Ms. Watkins represents a poor outcome of hospitalization. The following case studies highlight some of the challenges and opportunities for hospital staff to overcome these challenges during the course of treatment of isolated elders with dementia. The first case, Mr. Bates, represents a subgroup of isolated adults with AD for whom hospitalization presents the opportunity for evaluation and treatment leading to continued care in the community. The second case, Ms. Cannelli, represents a group for whom hospitalization represents the gateway to appropriate institutionalization.

Case Study: Mr. Bates

Mr. Bates is a 67-year-old Caucasian male who had lived in the Boston area his entire life. In contrast to Ms. Watkins, Mr. Bates appeared to have been isolated for most of his adult life, living alone in an apartment in South Boston. He was described by several informants as having been a loner much of his life, having few friends, never having married, and having no children. He had two brothers: one who lived in California, and another living in Rhode Island; and one sister who lived in a nursing home in the Boston area. Mr. Bates graduated from high school and worked in a bank until about age 60, though it is not clear in what role. He is described as having been "a character" and "odd" all of his life. There is no clear evidence of psychosis, no psychiatric hospitalizations, and he has not been diagnosed with schizophrenia.

Six years before we met Mr. Bates, he was hospitalized after being struck by a bus while crossing a busy street. He was not badly injured, but he stayed in the hospital for several days. This led to his having contact with social service personnel at the hospital where he was treated. The hospital social worker noticed his memory loss and made referrals to a senior home care agency for additional services, including Meals-on-Wheels, homemaker service, transportation, and assistance with medical appointments and medication. A follow-up evaluation with a neurologist was arranged, and Mr. Bates was subsequently diagnosed with "dementia" and began treatment with Aricept. His brother was invited to a meeting with professional staff serving Mr. Bates, and his clinical situation was explained. His brother subsequently became more involved, taking Mr. Bates to medical appointments and talking by phone with social service staff and physicians on a regular basis. His brother eventually stated that when Mr. Bates could no longer live in his apartment, he would invite Mr. Bates to live in his home.

Case Study: Ms. Cannelli

Ms. Cannelli was a 90-year-old Italian-American widowed woman who lived in Boston in the same house in which she raised her two children. She lived in a stable neighborhood with at least five first-degree relatives residing within a 20-mile radius. Her two children were busy professionals who did not have time to provide care and supervision. They were sufficiently distant enough to be unaware of their mother's predicament. Ms. Cannelli was described as having been a "very independent person" all of her life, someone who "always liked to do things on her own." She socialized primarily with family members and did not participate in many community organizations outside of her church. Her husband died 30 years ago, and she continued to rely on family for social contact and support. In the past 20 years, she rarely left her neighborhood and never had a driver's license.

Ms. Cannelli was recently hospitalized when she fell and broke her wrist. The hospital staff recognized her dementia and made referrals to the hospital's specialty dementia clinic. The family received education and support from the clinic staff. It became clear to all that Ms. Cannelli's dementia was too advanced for her to return home, and she was successfully placed in a special Alzheimer's long-term care unit. The transition was smooth, and Ms. Cannelli's safety and care were enhanced by the hospital staff's intervention.

STRATEGIES FOR WORKING WITH ISOLATED ADULTS WHO ARE HOSPITALIZED

Attend to Barriers to Entry

Pathways-to-care analyses (Knopman, Donohue, & Gutterman, 2000; Mellick, Gerhart, & Whiteneck, 2003; Rogler & Cortex, 1993) have been helpful in identifying barriers and supports to participation in health care faced by different groups of patients. A wide variety of barriers has been identified across groups and care settings. For example, for adults with Alzheimer's disease, difficulty recognizing the early symptoms and delays in getting a full evaluation are common barriers to the initiation of care (Boise, Morgan, Kaye, & Camicioli, 1999; Drebing, Laschever, Lyon, McCarty, Harden, & Herz, 2004).

When we examine isolated adults with AD, a range of new barriers becomes apparent. Alzheimer's disease impairs insight into their symptoms, compromising their ability to identify and get the help they need. In the cases described above, none of the patients with AD reported memory problems to hospital staff or to family or friends. For those who do recognize the need for services for dementia symptoms, additional barriers becomes apparent. Every clinical service has specific "entry" tasks that must be completed before someone can be admitted to the status of "patient." In most cases, people must travel to the care setting and provide basic information about what problem they are facing: Why they are there, evidence of insurance coverage or ability to pay, ability to provide basic background information such as age and address. Some care settings may require a referral from another provider, medical records, arranging appointments, and waiting in admissions areas. For adults with dementia with no family caregivers, even the smallest requirement can represent a substantial barrier to care.

We accompanied one of the participants in the VIP project to a hospital-based memory disorders clinic so that she could obtain a dementia work-up. After an anxious taxi ride in which she had to be reminded where we were going and why it was important for her to continue, we arrived in the admissions area of the hospital. Our participant was given two pages of forms to complete and asked to provide her insurance information. She was, of course, unable to complete these tasks without the active support of our staff. She was then told to report to the seventh floor for her evaluation. Guiding her through a maze of hallways and elevators, which she would never have been able to negotiate on her own, we eventually found the seventh floor location, only to discover that this was the wrong clinic. We returned to the admissions area to obtain the correct location, which was on the 4th floor. The patient was again given forms to fill out and asked to wait to see the neurologist. Again, we had to encourage the patient to remain in the waiting area, reminding her of why she was there and that it would be good to wait until she could see the doctor. By the time the neurologist invited the patient into the office, it was clear to us that it was highly unlikely that adults with even mild dementia could have passed through all of these challenges and arrived at the appointment without substantial help.

Attend to Communication

A key component of working with hospitalized patients with AD who live alone is to ensure the flow of communication about treatment and treatment compliance among medical providers, other professional providers, and informal caregivers in the community. When a nonisolated person is hospitalized, family caregivers typically play the role of the switchboard operator, channeling information from outside sources to hospital staff, and then from hospital staff back to everyone who provides support. This includes collecting data for providers about symptoms and compliance, sharing information from the provider to the rest of the family, and keeping everyone aware of what support each is providing and what ongoing problems remain unresolved. The provision of care is a team effort, and without that central caregiver, communication often breaks down with potentially disastrous results. In most cases, including those of Mr. Bates and Ms. Cannelli, we found that professionals in hospital settings had limited access to data because they had no informants who had any data themselves. Similarly, the key care providers for these adults were not aware of what inpatient clinicians were doing, and thus unable to support the discharge plan.

Gathering Clinical History

For inpatient clinical staff, as for researchers and other service providers, a key challenge is how to collect valid data to understand the situation. As with 50% of VIP participants, Ms. Cannelli and Mr. Bates were involved in ongoing outpatient treatments, and there were no apparent recognitions of memory impairment or dementia by their providers. It is clear that many clinicians were not adequately evaluating mental status and were not questioning the validity of the patients' reports. A more consistent screening of mental status or the use of simple screening measures such as the Mini-Mental Status Exam (MMSE) would greatly enhance the probability of recognizing an isolated patient with sufficient cognitive impairment to raise questions about his or her abilities to provide adequate clinical histories.

When it is clear that the patient's report is compromised, the hospital clinician must assess the accuracy of additional data available and identify other possible sources of information. We found that medical records often reflected the shared ignorance of the providers. While family contact with hospital staff may be limited, other valuable informants are available. For Mr. Bates, outpatient social service and resident staff for senior housing were invaluable sources of accurate information. These professionals are often involved on a daily basis with the patient and are motivated to provide information on behavioral issues, family involvement, and service agencies involved in the patient's care. They may also be able to identify additional informants—friends, neighbors, or other professionals who work closely with the individual. Hospital clinicians must be aggressive in seeking out these sources and recognize the impact of the patient's isolation and dementia on the data collected from these sources. We concluded that for this isolated group, we needed at least two, and preferably three, informants to get reasonably complete data. Given the inconsistent occurrence of safety incidents, for example, it seems likely that clinicians would want to utilize more than two informants.

Compensate for Lack of an Advocate

Family members who are active advocates for patients' care are not always perceived positively by hospitals and providers, sometimes because of unreasonable demands and sometimes because the demands require additional resources and changes in strategy that are not easily achieved. In one sense, isolated adults with dementia can be relatively easy to work with because they typically have no advocates. The physician or nursing staff are often the only people aware of their needs. The responsibility falls on the physician to act as the patient's advocate and to make the appropriate referrals for additional services. Unfortunately, inpatient providers do not always recognize this added responsibility with isolated adults, acting under the assumption that if the patient wants or needs something, he or she or a family member will speak up. The involvement of formal patient advocates on a regular basis may be one strategy to protect the patient and provider.

Successful Discharge Planning

Dealing with safety and legal issues with adults with dementia can be very challenging for providers, sometimes resulting in avoidance of the issue until pressed by family members. During the discharge planning process, providers work with family members to identify and address safety and legal issues. However, when there are no family members available, addressing safety and legal issues requires special attention. Following are some of the key safety and legal issues to address, and some suggestions for ways to approach them.

> *Driving and transportation.* In general, advising adults with dementia to cease driving is a formidable challenge; stopping someone who has no family may be even more difficult. Occupational

therapists who provide specialized driving assessment and other dementia and driving specialists are often experienced in this task and should be relied upon to provide guidance. Other providers, such as neighbors, family, and friends, can be enlisted. Those patients who use mass transit must be evaluated for the ability to do so safely and effectively. It was not uncommon for us to hear about VIP participants who were found by police in other parts of town, having traveled by subway, bus, or even walking to places they did not want to be and forgetting how to get home.

The home environment. Expectedly, the homes of VIP participants were dramatically different from the homes of other adults with dementia who live with caregivers. They were much more cluttered, dirty, disorganized, and unsafe. It was not uncommon to see rotting food in refrigerators and fire hazards around the home. Making a referral for a home visit is a critical step in evaluating whether the isolated adult can return safely to his or her home.

Medication errors. Some VIP participants were able to take their medications at home after they left the hospital, and some clearly could not do so without support. Of course, this ability depends in part on how many medications they were taking and the schedule. Some used pillboxes and other devices effectively, but others did not, a cause of anxiety for many providers. Referrals to adult daycare and in-home services were among the most common ways discharge plans effectively addressed concerns regarding medication.

Cooking. The clearest risk was for fire caused by cooking improperly or leaving the stove on after cooking was completed. In most cases where care providers became involved, the stove was permanently disabled and home-delivered meals were initiated, with reasonable success and safety.

Victimization. While the potential for victimization of isolated adults with dementia is high, we found few who clearly had been victimized among the VIP project participants. The most common pattern we found was a family member living with the VIP participant and using his or her resources, but contributing no support or resources.

Legal issues. There are several legal issues that should be assessed with all patients living alone with dementia. These include competency, the need for conservatorship and/or guardianship, the potential for eviction, the potential for victimization through abuse or neglect, and discrimination issues. During intake, it is important to assess whether the patient is the decision maker, and if so, is he or she competent enough to be making those decisions? It is important, therefore, to determine which players in the patient's social network may be able to take responsibility for decision making.

Strategies for Reducing Isolation

Building up existing informal supports and identifying potential supports. Hospital staff and other providers are in good positions to coordinate a plan that utilizes the patient's existing informal support network to provide effective support when the patient is discharged back home. We initially assumed that many of the adults in the VIP project would have long histories of isolation and would have little in the way of contacts that would be willing to get involved. To our surprise, we found that most participants had not been isolated for long periods of time. For many, isolation developed within the prior five years due to loss of family and friends to death and illness. We also found that almost all had some ongoing social contacts, whether with friends, neighbors, or family, who were willing to become more involved. Potential supports often do not understand the problems faced by the patient. Many understand part of the picture, but no one has asked them to help before. Potential supporters typically need information provided to them before they "buy into" getting involved. They need to learn about the illness, the isolation and risks involved, the elder's current and future needs, the other potential supports available, how much time and effort they will have to dedicate to caring for the elder, and the existing resources available to help them provide support. They often want to see that someone has a plan and to understand how they fit in. The plan must clearly and succinctly identify specific needs, specific steps, the person who is responsible for each step, a plan for follow-up, and revision as the situation changes.

Replace missing informal supports with formal supports. An alternative to developing informal supports is to substitute formal supports for them. This is a common strategy, as professional services are easier to initiate, and professional providers are often more consistently willing to be involved over time than informal supports. There is also a sense of shared clinical responsibility and liability that may be attractive to providers. Often, the patient without a family caregiver had already accrued a number of formal supports by the time his or her clinical providers become aware of and involved in dementia care. Hospital providers will want to survey which services are being received and for which services the participant is eligible. Formal supports, such as visiting nurses and adult day health programs in the patient's home area, can often help with treatment compliance. For the patient with dementia, private duty nurses and companions can help address safety concerns identified during the discharge planning stage and can be a resource for overnight supervision. Developing a pool of willing volunteers can further supplement supports for care and supervision.

CONCLUSIONS

The population of isolated elders with dementia is sizeable and growing. Current trends in modern culture, such as increased mobility, smaller number of offspring, and increased longevity, all suggest that the number of people living alone with AD is going to rise substantially. Hospital and community-based health care and social workers are at the front line of defense for this vulnerable population. While providing inpatient services to this isolated group can result in significant challenges, hospitalization can be a key decision point leading to more appropriate care for this group. Clinicians, administrators, and policymakers at both state and program levels must consider how best to address the needs of this group to ensure that, as a society, we provide for their care in a safe and effective manner.

REFERENCES

Alzheimer's Association. (2003). *NIA New: AD Research Update.* Retrieved August 18, 2003, from www.alzheimers.org/nianews/nianews59.html

Boise, L. Morgan. D. L., Kaye, J., & Camicioli, R. (1999). Delays in the diagnosis of dementia: Perspective of family caregivers. *American Journal of Alzheimer's Disease, 1,* 20–26.

Drebing, C. (1999). Trends in the content and methodology of Alzheimer's caregiving research. *Alzheimer's Disease and Related Disorders, 13*(S-1), S93–S100.

Drebing, C.E., Laschever, R., Lyon, P., McCarty, E., Harden, L. & Herz, L. (2004). Documenting Pathways to Care: Relative Validity of Questionnaire, Interview, and Medical Record Data. American Journal of Alzheimer's Disease and Other Dementias, 19 (3), 187–197.

Ebly, E. M., Hogan, D. B., & Rockwood, K. (1999). Living alone with dementia. *Dementia and Geriatric Cognitive Disorders, 10,* 541–548.

Fox, P. J., Lindeman, D. A., & Benjamin, A. E. (1988). *Evaluation of Alzheimer's disease diagnostic and treatment centers in California.* San Francisco, CA: University of California, Institute for Health and Aging.

Grossberg, G. T. (2003). Diagnosis and treatment of Alzheimer's disease. *Journal of Clinical Psychiatry, 64*(S9), 3–6.

Knopman, D., Donohue, J. A., & Gutterman, E. M. (2000). Patterns of care in the early stages of Alzheimer's disease: Impediments to timely diagnosis. *Journal of the American Geriatics Society, 48*(3), 300–304.

Leveist, T. A., Sellers, T. M., Brown, K. A., & Nickerson, K. J. (1998). Extreme social isolation, use of community-based senior support services, and mortality among African American elderly women. *American Journal of Community Psychology, 25,* 721–732.

Mellick, D., Gerhart, K. A., & Whiteneck, G. G. (2003). Understanding outcomes based on the post-acute hospitalization pathways followed by persons with traumatic brain injury. *Brain Injury, 17*(1), 49–54.

Minkler, M. (1986). Building support networks from social isolation. *Generations, 10*(4), 46–49.

Newhouse, B. J., Niebuhr, L., Stroud, T., & Newhouse, E. (2001). Living alone with dementia: Innovative support programs. *Alzheimer's Care Quarterly, 2*(2), 53–61.

Raschko, R. (1991). *Living alone with Alzheimer's disease: A social policy time bomb.* (Monograph).

Rathbone, M., E., & Hashimi, J. (1982). *Isolated elders: Health and social intervention.* Rockville, MD: Aspen Publications.

Rogler, L. H., & Cortex, D. E. (1993). Help-seeking pathways: A unifying concept in mental health care. *American Journal of Psychiatry, 150*(4), 554–560.

Steinback, U. (1992). Social networks, institutionalization, and mortality among elderly people in the United States. *Journals of Gerontology, 47*(4), S183–S190.

Tuokko, H., MacCourt, P., & Heath, T. (1999). Home alone with dementia. *Aging and Mental Health, 3*(1), 21–27.

U.S. Department of Health and Human Services. (1988). *Unpublished prevalence data from the Epidemiological Catchment Area Program.* Rockville, MD: National Institute of Mental Health, Epidemiology and Psychology Research Branch.

Webber, P. A., Fox, P., & Burnette, D. (1994). Living alone with Alzheimer's disease: Effects on health and social service utilization patterns. *Gerontologist, 34*(1), 8–14.

PART III

PROMISING APPROACHES FOR IMPROVING CARE FOR HOSPITALIZED ELDERS WITH DEMENTIA

Changing Dementia Care in a Hospital System

The Providence Milwaukie Experience

Frances Conedera and Jackie Beckwith

In 2001, Providence Milwaukie Hospital (PMH) began an ambitious project to improve care for patients with dementia. The dementia project was part of a larger effort by the the hospital to improve care for all its older patients. The project was supported by a grant from the Alzheimer's Association and involved a partnership with the local Alzheimer's Association. This chapter describes the dementia project at PMH, the rationale for the focus on dementia, and the philosophy of change that guided the project. The chapter identifies the aspects of care that were targeted for improvement in the dementia project, the specific activities implemented, and the practical obstacles encountered. Despite these obstacles, the project created and tested innovative ways of improving dementia care and resulted in valuable lessons for other hospitals seeking to improve the care they provide for patients with dementia.

PROVIDENCE MILWAUKIE HOSPITAL AND THE DECISION TO FOCUS ON DEMENTIA CARE

PMH is one of three hospitals operated by the Providence Health System (PHS) in the Portland, Oregon, metropolitan area. The PHS is a not-for-profit health care network that provides services in Oregon, Washington, Alaska, and California. PMH is a seventy-seven-bed community hospital that provides both inpatient and outpatient services. In 2000, PMH established an aggressive "Vision 2010" campaign to make the hospital a "Center of Excellence for Aging."

The area surrounding the hospital mirrors the U.S. population, with about 13% of community residents in the 65 and older age group. In 2000, PMH had 3,400 admissions, 45% of which were people aged 65 and older. Older hospital patients have multiple health care needs that are impacted by complications related to aging (Abraham, Bottrell, Fulmer, & Mezey, 1999). In its "Vision 2010," PMH leadership focused on identification and development of health care services and delivery systems that would meet the special needs of an aging population.

"Vision 2010" was a part of a larger effort in the Portland Area PHS to improve hospital care for all older patients. Toward this end, each hospital became part of "Nurses Improving Care for Health System Elders" (NICHE), a national program of the John A. Hartford Institute for Geriatric Nursing at New York University. NICHE is a nurse-driven program intended to provide nurses with tools and expertise to develop excellence in practice for elderly patients. Like many hospitals that affiliate with the national NICHE program, PMH referred to its own program to improve care for elderly patients as NICHE, of which the dementia project was a part.

One component of the national NICHE program is an organizational assessment, called the Geriatric Institutional Assessment Profile (GIAP). The GIAP instrument includes questions about staff knowledge of geriatric practice and staff perceptions of the quality of geriatric care and the milieu for geriatric practice in their institutions. In addition, questions address the level of difficulty staff experiences in caring for elderly patients, which patient behaviors are most disturbing, and whether staff members have confidence in their ability to manage these behaviors.

The GIAP is generally administered only to nursing staff. PMH administered the tool to a broader group of patient care staff members; Figure 8.1 shows results from the GIAP assessment. More than half of the PMH staff members who completed the GIAP reported problems with elderly patients who wander during the day, and about one-third reported problems with elderly patients who are up at night. The percentage of staff reporting other problems was even higher. Elders who are uncooperative (70%), confused and agitated (68%), argumentative (61%), or demanding (58%) posed significant challenges for staff. Nurses in particular found these behaviors troublesome because they often occurred at night or during the busy evening shift and frequently resulted in use of restraints or psychotropic medications.

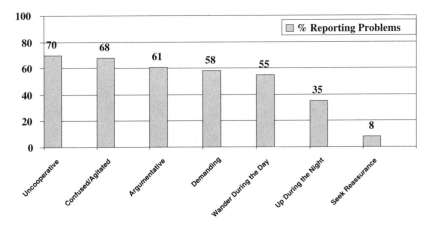

FIGURE 8.1   Percentage of PMH staff reporting problems with behavior of older patients, Geriatric Institutional Assessment Profile, Sept. 2000.

Although any hospital patient may be argumentative, demanding, or up during the night, other behaviors reported as difficult by PMH staff (wandering, uncooperative, confused and agitated) are more likely to occur in patients with dementia. These GIAP findings were a major factor in the PMH decision to focus on dementia.

As noted earlier, PMH conducted its dementia project in the context of its "Vision 2010" and NICHE efforts. Thus, the hospital was simultaneously trying to improve dementia care, and geriatric care in general, all under the umbrella of its NICHE program.

PHILOSOPHY OF CHANGE

Theories about how change occurs are valuable when trying to create change. The "Transtheoretical Model for Change" (Prochaska, Johnson, & Lee, 1998) describes five stages of change:

1. *Pre-contemplation:* the stage in which the possibility of change is considered;
2. *Contemplation:* the stage in which there is awareness that a problem exists and consideration of change, but no commitment to take action;
3. *Preparation:* the stage in which there is a stated commitment to change;
4. *Action:* the stage in which modifications of behaviors are initiated; and

5. *Maintenance:* the stage in which people work to prevent relapse and consolidate gain.

Within this model of change, PMH was in the contemplation stage at the beginning of the dementia project.

To create change, it would be necessary to develop both commitment and a clear plan of action. The work of William Bridges (1998) was useful in understanding and evaluating the organization and the nursing unit's readiness for change. Bridges (1998) also provides specific strategies for managing change and guiding staff through multiple, concurrent changes.

The philosophy of change underlying PMH's planning for the dementia project and concurrent work with geriatric care in general included beliefs about the importance of the following factors for a successful change process:

- *Attention to staff attitudes as well as care protocols.* Change would require the development of patient care protocols to guide care of hospitalized elders, including those with dementia. In addition, however, it was necessary to recognize pervasive, negative societal attitudes toward elders, especially those with dementia. Nurses and other hospital staff share some of these negative societal attitudes. Following best-practice protocols that demonstrate a decrease or better management of "problems" with elders could result in change in attitudes among providers.
- *An interdisciplinary approach.* Leadership of NICHE was assumed by nursing. Nursing spends the majority of the hospital stay with patients; the national NICHE program is led by nurses, and nursing is in the best position to develop and implement care protocols. At the same time, many other hospital disciplines, including social services, respiratory therapy, physical therapy, pastoral care, pharmacy, nutritional therapy, and medicine would need to participate actively for change to occur.
- *Involvement of all levels of staff.* Abraham, Bottrell, Fulmer, and Mezey (1999) argue that mixed groups of physicians, nurses, and other patient care staff found in hospital units will have the greatest chance of success in creating change. The participation of project leaders, mid-level managers, and staff members encourages "buy-in" and therefore an acceptance and willingness to adapt to change. Staff consensus and a sense of ownership are seen as the best predictors of successful adoption and maintenance of practice change.

- *Focus on motivation.* Would nurses and other patient care staff change their usual care practices if they were told it was the "right" thing to do, or if they became more aware of the large number of elderly patients and patients with dementia in the hospital? Would the GIAP findings influence staff care practices? Would the fact that the GIAP results were identified by staff affect staff behavior? All of these factors would influence change. Francis and Bottrell (1999) say that nurses will adopt changes in practice more readily if the problem is a problem for them, if the changes are proven and clearly outlined, and if they believe the changes will help them care for their patients. Social influence theory argues that choices directing decisions and actions are affected by the habits, customs, beliefs, and values of peers. Prevailing practice, social norms, and economic concerns also influence how individual nurses and other patient care staff evaluate and potentially adopt new practice information (Abraham et al., 1999). Over the years, nursing encounters with patients have evolved to brief, sometimes superficial, interactions. Even with nurse-to-patient ratios of 1:3 or 1:4, interactions have become limited to providing merely the essentials of care (Kitwood, 1999). Clearly, it would take more than information and the GIAP findings to change staff attitudes and care practices for elderly patients and patients with dementia, and then, ultimately, to turn the staff into active advocates for this patient population.

A carefully orchestrated step-by-step process was needed to develop best-practice delivery of care and overcome resistance to change. This plan included:

1. Creation of a team to implement change
2. Adequate supervision and guidance to the goals
3. A plan for staff development and training
4. A process for accreditation and promotion
5. Effective quality monitors

In 2000, an interdisciplinary steering committee was appointed to implement this process and oversee PMH's NICHE program. The steering committee focused first on creating a desire or motivation on the part of the staff to adopt improvements in their care practices. Concise, practice-based processes, tools, procedures, and standards of care were the next priority.

BEGINNINGS OF THE DEMENTIA PROJECT

The GIAP findings were a major factor in the PMH decision to focus on dementia. Nurses and other patient care staff had identified their concerns about care of patients with dementia and their need for knowledge and skill development in this area. Some staff members also expressed a need for information about community referrals for these patients.

Through the Providence Center on Aging, a partnership with the local Alzheimer's Association Chapter was established. In late 2000, the national Alzheimer's Association issued a request for letters of intent for a pilot project to improve hospital care for people with dementia. One of the requirements for submission was a strong partnership between the hospital and an Alzheimer's Association Chapter. That partnership already existed through the Center on Aging and the Oregon Trails Chapter of the Alzheimer's Association. The PMH project was chosen as the grant recipient in spring 2001.

Aspects of Care Targeted for Improvement in the Dementia Project

Initially, five aspects of hospital care for people with dementia were targeted:

1. *Recognition of cognitive impairment/dementia at the time of admission and collection of patient information to support care planning:* Procedures would be developed to assess cognitive function in elderly patients on admission. Information about the patients' prehospital sleep patterns, mobility, attention, speech, mood, and need for hearing and vision aids would serve as a baseline for planning their hospital care.
2. *Identification of special risks and needs:* Training would be provided to help staff identify patients with dementia who are at risk. These risks might include falls, increased cognitive impairment, polypharmacy, and increased functional impairment. Referrals to other disciplines were anticipated to increase.
3. *Use of nonpharmacological interventions:* At least one nonpharmacological intervention would be identified and used to maintain or improve prehospital functioning for each patient with dementia.
4. *Involvement of families in discharge planning:* Staff would work with patients' families throughout patients' hospital stays to develop discharge plans. Such plans would continue the pre-

hospital and hospital interventions aimed at maintaining patient functioning.

5. *Dementia information and education for patients' families:* The Alzheimer's Association Chapter would conduct dementia information sessions in the hospital and provide printed materials for distribution in the hospital.

Expansion of Focus to Include the 3 Ds: Dementia, Delirium, and Depression

The project steering committee decided to add delirium and depression to the original focus of dementia. One reason for this decision was the difficulty of differentiating these three conditions in elderly hospital patients, especially at the time of admission. In addition, dementia is a strong risk factor for delirium, and greater staff awareness of both conditions and their interrelationship could result in proactive interventions that might prevent or reduce an episode of delirium (Foreman, Trygstad, & Fletcher, 2003). Lastly, chart reviews showed that elderly patients with cognitive impairment who acknowledged depression on admission often received no further assessment or intervention. As a result of the steering committee decision, differentiation of dementia, delirium, and depression was identified as a basic learning objective for all disciplines providing patient care.

INNOVATIVE ACTIVITIES IMPLEMENTED IN THE DEMENTIA PROJECT

From May 2001 to early 2003, PMH instituted ten new activities that were expected to improve dementia care. Some of the activities, especially early on, addressed dementia in the larger context of geriatric care, while later activities focused more specifically on dementia. Changes were implemented on the medical surgical unit and in the ICU.

The ten activities are described below in the order in which they were first instituted, although some were repeated one or more times over the project period.

1. *Kick-Off for the NICHE Program.* In November 2001, the steering committee hosted a hospital-wide event to introduce the NICHE program. All hospital staff members were invited. "Stations" were set up for staff to experience the effects of impairments that are common with aging. These included: vision and

hearing impairments, loss of tactile sensation, and mobility problems. There was a debriefing discussion regarding the experiential activities and staff learning.

2. *Patient Care Rounds.* In May 2001, multidisciplinary patient care rounds were instituted on the hospital's medical surgical unit. The rounds were conducted once a week, focusing on "difficult" patients or those who met preestablished criteria. Often, although not always, the focus was patients with dementia, delirium, and/or depression and related care issues, such as behavioral problems, medications, pain management, and discharge planning. The weekly rounds resulted in rich discussions among all disciplines, generating more questions and interventions and increasing staff awareness of special risks and needs associated with dementia along with the importance of follow-up and family involvement. A striking characteristic of the patient care rounds was the regular attendance of most disciplines. Results of the rounds were:
   • Increased referrals to disciplines other than nursing
   • Thoughtful and timely discharge planning
   • Intentional discussions with family members regarding specific care or discharge issues
   • Identification of ethical issues for referral to the hospital's ethics committee
   • Review of patient medications with a discussion of interactions, side effects, and medication alternatives for consideration by the patient's physician

3. *3 Ds Intensive Training for Nurses.* In December 2001, an eight-hour educational program for nurses was presented by faculty from the OHSU School of Nursing. The training curriculum included segments on normal cognition in older people; mental status assessment; the etiology, symptoms, and usual course of dementia, delirium, depression, grief, and bereavement; challenging nursing dilemmas in dementia care; and environmental, psychosocial, and pharmacological interventions useful in management of dementia-related behavioral symptoms. This eight-hour program was repeated in April 2002 and July 2002, and parts of it were later incorporated into PMH training for newly hired nurses.

4. *Informational Sessions and Materials for Families.* In January 2002, the Alzheimer's Association Chapter sponsored a series of four informational meetings for families at the hospital. The four-meeting series, "Living with Alzheimer's Disease," included

sessions on the definition, course, and treatment of Alzheimer's disease; techniques for minimizing communication and behavioral problems; legal and financial issues; and community resources. Each session was attended by fifteen to thirty family members, most of whom were adult daughters of people with dementia. The Chapter also provided print materials about Alzheimer's disease and dementia that were placed in display racks in public areas of the hospital. These materials disappeared quickly and had to be replenished often.

5. *Revision of the Hospital's Admission Assessment Form.* The PMH admission assessment form asks about Alzheimer's, dementia, and confusion. In 2002, additional items were added to help staff identify patients with dementia (See Fig. 8.2).

   Positive responses to the "confusion" item and the questions about cognitive function do not indicate a diagnosis of dementia but rather a need for further assessment of the patient's cognitive status. Other sections of the assessment form included questions about depression and areas of special concern for patients with dementia, e.g., activities of daily living, recent falls, mobility problems, pain, swallowing difficulties, and use of dentures, glasses, and hearing aids. This information supported the development of standardized care plans that could be individualized to address the special risks and needs of patients.

6. *Procedures for Further Assessment of Patients with Possible Dementia.* A literature search led to selection of the Mini Mental Status Exam (MMSE) and the Geriatric Depression Scale (GDS) as instruments to be used for further assessment. The limitations of these instruments are well known (Butler, Lewis, &

Prior to this admission, have you experienced problems in:

Cognitive Function ____ Yes* ____ No Describe _____
(i.e., able to talk, write, read, and follow directions, adequate memory or recall)

Special equipment used to assist you with communicating? ____ Yes* ____ No

a. Are familiar activities sometimes difficult to complete? ____ Yes* ____ No
b. Do familiar places sometimes seem unfamiliar? ____ Yes* ____ No
c. Have you experienced recent, frequent mood swings that surprise you?
    ____ Yes* ____ No

*Follow up required.

FIGURE 8.2   Questions about cognitive function on the admission assessment form, Providence Milwaukie Hospital, 2001.

Sunderland, 1998). The advantages include ease of staff training, widespread use with validity and reliability for many patient
populations, and minimal time for completion.

Once the two instruments were selected, criteria were established for their use: The MMSE would be used for all patients
aged 75 and older; any patient with the item "dementia/Alzheim-
er's" or "confusion" circled on his or her admission assessment
form; any patient with a positive response to the questions about
cognitive function on the assessment form; and any patient referred for assessment by a physician. The GDS would be used
for all patients with a positive response to the question about
depression on the admission form; patients with other specified
symptoms; and patients referred for assessment by a physician.[1]

A two-hour training program on the use and interpretation
of both the MMSE and GDS was offered multiple times and in
new employee orientation. A video demonstration provided by
the Alzheimer's Association offered immediate practice and feedback. Staff members were encouraged to contact the hospital's
nurse educator for help the first few times they did the assessments, until they felt comfortable with this new skill.

Electronic medical records provided data regarding use of
the MMSE and GDS. A printout was generated every day showing the names of all inpatients aged 75 and older. The printout
also showed the number of MMSE and GDS assessments that
had been completed in the previous 24 hours, the names of the
patients who were assessed, and the name of the nurse who did
the assessment. Use of the MMSE and GDS was very limited at
first. Some nurses were concerned about the time involved in
completing the assessments, but other nurses reported only five
to ten minutes for completion. In unit meetings and one-on-one
conversations, project leaders and nurse managers encouraged
nurses to do the assessments and praised nurses who completed
them.

7. *New Standard of Care for Cognitive Impairment/Dementia.* In
   July 2002, the new standard of care for dementia was introduced.
   A standard of care (SOC) is a formal document intended to guide

---

[1]Despite the steering committee's decision to expand the dementia project to include the
3 Ds, no instrument was selected for further assessment of delirium. The main reason for
this was lack of agreement between PMH and its sister hospitals about which instrument
would be best and exactly what interventions should be used to treat delirium. In addition,
introduction of three new instruments at one time had little chance of success.

nursing care. PMH developed its Standard of Care for Cognitive Impairment/Dementia on the basis of staff knowledge and information from a nursing text by Maas, Tripp-Reimer, Buckwalter, and Titler. (2001). The SOC identifies six goal areas: (1) maximizing safe function; (2) providing patients with unconditional positive regard; (3) recognizing patient behaviors, such as anxiety and avoidance, as indicators that the level of activity and stimulation is too high for the patient; (4) "listening" to the patient, with attention to both verbal and nonverbal communications; (5) modifying the environment to minimize losses and enhance safety; and (6) providing ongoing education, support, and problem-solving assistance for family caregivers. In each goal area, the SOC lists two to ten nonpharmacological interventions that could be used to achieve the goal. The goals and interventions included in the SOC were discussed in the 3 Ds educational program, which was presented twice before the standard of care was introduced and again in July 2002. An additional 2-hour class focused on the correlation of the admission assessment, patient care planning, and the SOC. Admission assessments indicating possible dementia would trigger further assessment of cognitive status and the development of patient care plans that reflected the goals and interventions outlined in the SOC. This sequence of activities would allow nurses to provide care for patients with dementia in an intentional way that recognized the special risks and needs caused by the patients' dementia.

8. *Referral Information for the Alzheimer's Association Chapter's 24-hour Hotline.* In July 2002, the Chapter's 24-hour hotline was introduced with written pocket cards for families and staff.

9. *Activity Kits for Patients with Dementia.* In August 2002, activity kits for patients with dementia were introduced on the medical-surgical and critical care units. PMH staff worked with rehabilitation personnel from a sister hospital to develop the kits. Both functional and cognitive abilities were considered in selecting the activity kit items. The kits contain pegboards, small geometric puzzles, stacking cones, magazines, playing cards, tapes, and CDs. Combination radio, tape, and CD players were purchased and made available for patient use.

The activity kits were intended to provide stimulation and diversion, reduce boredom, agitation, and resulting behavioral problems, and ultimately avoid the use of physical restraints and medications to manage these problems. It was not possible to quantify use of the kits, but anecdotal reports indicated that they

were being used on the two units. Staff also made helpful suggestions about items that could be added to the kits.[2]

10. *Chapter Information for Physicians Added to Hospital Packets
    for New Residents.* In January 2003, the Alzheimer's Associa-
    tion Chapter's information packet for physicians was added to
    the orientation materials for new PMH medical residents.

In addition to the ten activities described above, in-service training
programs on topics related to dementia care were presented at PMH
during the project period. These programs included four in-services on
disruptive patients, an in-service on medications for sedation in critical
care, and an in-service on alternatives to physical restraints.

EVALUATION OF THE DEMENTIA PROJECT

Quantitative approaches were used to evaluate the eight-hour training
program on the 3 Ds to determine how often the MMSE, GDS, and
SOC were implemented, and to identify changes in the extent to which
symptoms of dementia and interventions for dementia were noted in patient charts. The 8-hour training program began with a pre-test. Three
months later, the same test was sent out to nurses who had participated
in the training. The return rate was minimal in spite of two reminder notices and the offer of an incentive for those who completed and returned
the test. The resulting numbers were too small to capture meaningful
data about retention.

As noted earlier, each time an MMSE or GDS was completed, staff
members were instructed to record it in the computer. The resulting computer records showed very few completed assessments. Likewise, a chart
audit for a sample of fifty patients aged 75 and over that was conducted
in October 2002 by OHSU nursing students found only three charts
with documented MMSE and GDS assessments and only two charts that
contained the new SOC form. Moreover, hospital discharge data for the
one-year period from October 2001 to October 2002 showed no change
in the proportion of elderly patients who were discharged with a primary or secondary ICD-9 code diagnosis of dementia.

---

[2]Ideas developed for this project about activity kits are included in *"Try This: Therapeutic
Activity Kits"* by Frances Conedera and Laura Mitchell. The *Try This* series includes brief
training documents for hospital nurses (see Chapter 12).

In contrast, other findings from the October 2002 chart audit suggest considerable improvement in recognition of dementia and use of dementia-related interventions. Findings from the October 2002 chart audit were compared with findings from a similar chart audit that was conducted in October 2001 (before the first 3 Ds training program, changes in the admission assessment form, and introduction of the MMSE, GDS, and SOC). This comparison indicates that over the one-year period, recognition of cognitive impairment in elderly patients at the time of hospital admission increased from 4% to 38%, and recognition of cognitive impairment in elderly patients at any time during hospitalization increased from 34% to 62%. Documentation of interventions to address memory problems, communication issues, safety, toileting, nutrition, and family involvement also increased, although without explicit reference to the SOC.

The October 2002 chart audit shows increased use of two types of medications that are sometimes prescribed for management of agitation and behavioral problems in people with dementia. Specifically, use of antipsychotics increased from 6% to 14%, and use of benzodiazepenes increased from 2% to 24%. Information from the chart audit is not sufficient to evaluate the appropriateness of this increase in use. It is possible that increased recognition of dementia led to increased use of the medications, even though the training programs for the dementia project emphasized the importance of trying nonpharmacological approaches first and avoiding use of these types of medications whenever possible.

Comparison of the chart audits for October 2001 and October 2002 also shows that recognition of depression in elderly patients at the time of hospital admission increased 6% to 28%. There was no change, however, in the use of antidepressant medications.

Considered together, these evaluation findings present a mixed picture. On the positive side, there was increased recognition of dementia and depression and increased use of dementia-related interventions. Yet, there was little evidence that the tools for further assessment and care planning (the MMSE, GDS, and SOC) were being used. The second chart audit was conducted only three months after the SOC was introduced and ten months after the first dementia training. At this writing, the October 2003 audit demonstrates a significant increase in use of the MMSE. However, the data also demonstrate lack of attention to the established criteria for patient selection and minimal use of the SOC for patients identified with dementia. This seems to indicate an increased awareness by staff members that the MMSE is required but a lack of understanding regarding the indicators for its use and application.

OBSTACLES TO IMPLEMENTATION

Bridges (1998) recommends that during an attempt to make a major shift in their practices and culture, organizations limit unnecessary changes. However some changes or external factors are not always in the researchers' control. This was the case with the PMH project. It is important to mention the obstacles encountered, should such changes be tried in other hospital settings.

In the same period as the dementia project, multiple changes were occurring at PMH. These changes diverted staff attention and resources from the project and created significant obstacles to implementation. Changes with the greatest impact on the project's implementation included the following:

- *Protracted union negotiations:* In December 2001, for the first time in PMH history, registered nurses voted to join a union. Contract negotiations lasted for two years. Following mediation, a tentative agreement was reached with the nurses in November 2003. Ratification of the contract occurred by December 2003. Contract negotiations were disruptive, in part because preexisting conflicts that separated management and staff were magnified. Such disruptions often inhibited enthusiastic involvement in the project by all levels of staff, a factor believed essential for success.
- *JCAHO survey:* In late 2001, the Joint Commission on Accreditation of Healthcare Organizations (JCAHO) announced that it would conduct a routine but extensive survey at PMH in September 2002. In theory, hospitals are prepared at all times for such surveys; however, most hospitals spend the months preceding the visit in intense preparation. Such preparations include meetings, chart reviews and audits, creation or revision of forms, and staff preparation. At PMH, department managers were assigned responsibility for a set of JCAHO standards, which required a modification of priorities. This proved a distraction from the dementia project.
- *Computerization of patient records:* In 2002, PMH began a phased transition from a paper to computerized documentation system. This was a major change that involved training sessions, "go-live" dates, feedback, and modification of record-keeping processes.

Staffing issues also created obstacles for the dementia project. Nursing shortages plague hospitals across the nation, and PMH is no exception. Shortages result in a higher than usual use of on-call and agency personnel who may not know of or be committed to long-term hospital projects. The medical-surgical nurse manager position at PMH proved difficult to fill, and the dementia project was underway for six months before a manager was hired. Unfilled positions can result in fragmented project leadership, and missed opportunities for teaching, mentoring, and bedside modeling of assessment procedures and recommended interventions.

The Alzheimer's Association Chapter also experienced organizational and staffing problems that interfered with implementation of dementia project activities. The Chapter's long-time executive director, who had taken a strong interest in the project, retired in June 2002, and the Chapter staff member who had provided focus on the project left the Chapter at about the same time. The new executive director could not give immediate attention to the project, and the staff member assigned to the project had many other responsibilities. Consequently, the Chapter was unable to follow through on some planned activities, including a series of family informational meetings about late-stage Alzheimer's disease planned for the summer of 2002 and a repetition of the January 2002 informational meeting that was planned for later in the year.

It is unclear whether some of these obstacles could have been avoided or their effects reduced. Bridges (1998) advises that when an organization plans to make major changes, it should evaluate the impact of the changes on the overall organizational processes as well as include in the evaluation the impact each change would have on others. In doing so, a plan can be developed to manage the whole as well as each separate change. This advice applies to changes that are anticipated and planned, but many of the changes that created obstacles for the dementia project could not have been anticipated. Difficulties with staffing at PMH and the Alzheimer Association Chapter might have been anticipated but probably could not have been avoided. The cumulative effect of unexpected changes and staffing problems slowed implementation of project activities and made the project more difficult to administer. Consequently, some of the planned activities were delayed, a few were eliminated from the plan, and project momentum was significantly diminished, at least in the short term.

ONGOING ISSUES

In the context of the five-stage model of change cited earlier (Prochaska et al., 1998), PMH had clearly moved from contemplation through the preparation stage and was well into the action stage by the end of the dementia project. As previously noted, in the action stage, behavior modification has begun, but a significant commitment of time and energy is still needed by participants. Successful navigation through behavioral change leads the project to the fifth stage in the model: the maintenance stage, in which activities are focused on preventing relapse and consolidating the group's gains. Efforts to maintain the integrity of the NICHE program, to prevent relapse, and to consolidate the gains of improved care for all geriatric patients at PMH included providing staff support for progressive change, development of adequate assessment tools, and formulation of a valid evaluation process to document progress. It was determined that focused efforts should include:

- *Ongoing staff training, access to expert clinical advice, and opportunities for practice-level discussion:* Training provided through the dementia project was well received, and chart audits suggest that it had a positive effect. Efforts by nurses and other care staff to comply with the changes were apparent; however, the attrition rate for the medical-surgical unit was high, and training needed to be repeated regularly. Availability of clinical experts to answer questions, help refine interventions, and conduct patient care rounds would reinforce learning. In September 2004, a clinical development specialist position was created to manage education and quality improvement. This position could significantly impact continuous clinical training.
- *Analysis of the limited use of the MMSE, GDS, and SOC, incorporating needed revisions:* It is not clear why the two assessment instruments and SOC were initially used so infrequently. Perhaps patient and family education, collaboration with medical staff, support for ongoing progress, and its *meaning* for improved geriatric care would be reflected in improved compliance with the tools. Careful analysis of the reasons for limited use of the tools might determine whether different assessment instruments or revisions to the SOC would encourage better compliance.
- *Dementia information and education for families:* The Alzheimer's Association sponsored a four-week series of informational meetings for families and provided printed material to be displayed in racks throughout the hospital. Informational meetings should be repeated often, and the display racks should be restocked regularly to keep information available for families.
- *Physician involvement:* The dementia project was structured to involve physicians along with all other direct care staff in the hospital. However, physician participation was minimal. Creative ways to encourage physician participation should be developed.

- *Continued efforts to improve geriatric care:* The dementia project was conducted in the context of a larger effort to improve care for all elderly patients. It is believed that better care for patients with dementia must be built on a foundation of good geriatric care. PMH and the Portland-area division of PHS have made significant inroads in improving geriatric care. A regional certification preparation course was developed to prepare and support PHS nurses for national certification in geriatric nursing. A need was identified for nurses to champion, mentor, teach by example, and take a leadership role in geriatric care with all hospital disciplines. Two PMH nurses were selected to assume this role. A Geriatric Resource Team was established to assume responsibility for encouraging and facilitating improvements in hospital care for elderly patients. Administrative support for all these activities will serve to improve geriatric and dementia care and provide a strong foundation for continued improvements.

One of the five aspects of care targeted for change at the beginning of the dementia project was family involvement in discharge planning. Discharge planning has always been a priority for nursing, but families are often not sufficiently involved. Incorporating family participation in assessing and collaborating on relatives' needs during hospitalization is the ideal. Best practice should result in discharge plans that help to maintain the patient's optimal health and functioning. The dementia project did not progress as far as discharge planning, and further work is needed on this aspect of care. Part of effective discharge planning for patients with dementia is connecting them and their families with their local Alzheimer's Association Chapter. The project provided wallet-size cards for staff and brochures for families with information about the Chapter's 24-hour hotline, but additional procedures should be developed to ensure that these connections occur. Nursing staff proposed to conduct post-discharge telephone calls with patients and families to discern their perceptions about the quality of geriatric care provided in the hospital. These discharge-related activities have not been developed and should be addressed.

A final issue is to develop a support structure for families while the patient is still in the hospital. Providing such support was an objective for PMH and the Alzheimer Association Chapter. People with dementia often have other serious medical conditions, and dementia is usually not the main reason they are hospitalized. Moreover, current hospital stays are very short. In the period of the dementia project, the average length of stay for PMH patients aged 65 and over ranged from 3.2 to 3.5 days. Discharge data for the year 2000 indicate an even shorter average length of stay (2.6 days) for patients with a discharge diagnosis of dementia. Given these very short hospital stays and the necessity to focus first on the primary reason for the patient's admission, it is often difficult for staff to find time to explore with families their dementia-related concerns.

CONCLUSION

The dementia project met its goal to develop and test activities intended to improve care for patients with dementia. Because there has been little previous work in this area, the experience at PMH provides valuable information for other hospitals interested in similar projects. The partnerships PMH developed with the Association Chapter and the division of nursing at a nearby academic medical center were helpful in planning and implementing the project. Use of the GIAP was helpful in identifying problems from the perspective of direct care staff. Decisions made by the steering committee, for example, the decision to conduct the dementia project in the larger context of geriatric care and to focus on dementia as one of the 3 Ds, reflect important insights about the role of dementia in the organizational and practice environment of hospitals.

Some activities that were implemented in the project were successful while others were not. Changes made to the admission assessment form targeted to increase recognition of dementia in the patient population seemed to work well. In contrast, the MMSE, GDS, and SOC were utilized infrequently.

Many activities were tried. It is unclear whether the project would have been more successful if it had attempted fewer activities, or conversely, whether this more comprehensive array of activities was more likely to be effective. While the dementia project was successful in many ways, much remains to be done. Many unanticipated changes and staffing problems interfered with carefully developed project plans and timelines and may have limited the effectiveness of some activities. Such changes and staffing problems should be anticipated in any future projects of this kind, and time should be built in to accommodate them.

There is no guarantee that the improvements in dementia care practices that were made at PMH will last. Any attempt to implement and maintain change will require ongoing support from senior management. This support must be active in word, role modeling, and resource allocation. Staying in touch with the change effort, asking for presentations in public forums, acknowledging both successes and problems, and checking on resource utilization all elevate the importance of the effort and therefore its likelihood of success. A small hospital such as PMH provides an ideal setting to garner active support from senior management.

Making rounds, talking to direct-care staff, and asking about project progress take minimal time in a weekly or monthly schedule. Activities such as these demonstrate the hospital's commitment to change and reinforce to direct care staff that what they are trying to do matters, which is the only way meaningful and lasting improvements in care will occur.

REFERENCES

Abraham, I., Bottrell, M., Fulmer, T., & Mezey, M. (Eds.) (1999). *Geriatric nursing protocols for best practice.* New York: Springer.

Bridges, W. (1998). *Facilitator guide: Leading organizational transition.* (Available from William Bridges & Associates, 38 Miller Avenue, Suite 12, Mill Valley, CA, 94941.)

Butler, R., Lewis, M., & Sunderland, T. (1998). *Aging and mental health: Positive psychosocial and biomedical approaches* (5th ed.). Boston: Allyn & Bacon.

Conedera, F., & Mitchell, L. (2004). Therapeutic activity kits. *Try this* from The John A. Hartford Institute for Geriatric Nursing. Available: www.hartfordign.org

Foreman, M., Mion, L., Trygstad, L., & Fletcher, K. (2003). Delirium: strategies for assessing and treating. In M. Mezey, T. Fulmer, & I. Abraham (Eds.). *Geriatric protocols for best practice* (pp. 116–140). New York: Springer.

Francis D., Bottrell M., & The NICHE Faculty. (1999). Implementing clinical practice protocols: Translating knowledge into practice. In I. Abraham, M. Botrell, T. Fulmer, and M. Mezey (Eds.), *Geriatric nursing protocols for best practice* (pp. 199–220). New York: Springer.

Kitwood, T. (1999). *Dementia reconsidered: The person comes first* (Rev. ed.). Buckingham, England: Open University Press.

Maas, M., Tripp-Reimer, T., Buckwalter, K.C., & Titler, A.G. (2001). *Nursing care of older adults: Diagnoses, outcomes, and interventions.* St. Louis: Mosby.

Prochaska, J.O., Johnson, S., & Lee, P. (1998). The transtheoretical model for change. In S. Shumaker, and E. B. Schron (Eds.), *The handbook of health behavior change* (2nd ed., pp. 58–84.). New York: Springer.

CHAPTER NINE

A NICHE Delirium Prevention Project for Hospitalized Elders

Patricia Finch Guthrie, Susan Schumacher, and Germaine Edinger

Preexisting dementia has been identified as a predisposing factor for delirium in hospitalized elders (Inouye & Charpentier, 1996). With the incidence of delirium documented as high as 56% for elders (Inouye, Schlesinger, & Lydon, 1999; Marcantonio, Flacker, Wright, & Resnick, 2001) and with the expected increase in the number of older adults with Alzheimer's disease and other dementias (Sparks, 2001), the hospital delirium rate may continue to increase if delirium prevention is not incorporated into routine care. Because delirium has been associated with poor outcomes (Inouye et al. 1999), it behooves hospital administrators to support clinicians in providing safe, vigilant geriatric care.

In 1998, the patient care services division at North Memorial Health Care (NMHC) participated in a Nurses Improving Heath System Elders (NICHE) conference at New York University. Through the faculty's guidance and one year of planning, NMHC started a NICHE program in 1999 and named the program, "Together We Improve Care of Elders" (TWICE). A goal for the TWICE program was an interdisciplinary focus instead of developing strictly a nursing program for improving geriatric care. Thus, an interdisciplinary steering committee was created to guide the program.

NMHC is a 400-bed, community-based level one trauma center in Robbinsdale, a suburb of Minneapolis, Minnesota. Like many hospitals, NMHC's patient population has shifted toward older and sicker patients with 30% of patients being 70 years or older. The average length of stay for older patients at NMHC is 4.5 days compared to 4.2 days for patients in all age groups. The most common diagnoses for elders are pneumonia, hip fracture, and major joint replacement. Due to physicians' inconsistent documentation of delirium as a discharge diagnosis in the medical record, delirium is not accurately captured in hospital administrative data. This is a common problem for acute care settings, which makes it difficult to determine actual delirium rates without conducting prospective studies or retrospective chart reviews (Kirkland, 1995). In a 1998 NMHC study on a medical-surgical unit and a cardiovascular unit, the delirium rates were found to be high for older patients (age 70 and older; 31%, n = 118 and 26%, n = 113, respectively). An innovative approach to improve care was needed, even though hospital statistics did not demonstrate that delirium was a significant problem. In this chapter, we describe the unit-based approach for preventing and managing delirium and the progression to an organization-based model. Both are NICHE models that can decrease the incidence of delirium.

INITIATING THE TWICE PROGRAM

An initial step for developing the TWICE program at NMHC was to form a steering committee that included administrators, multiple disciplines, gerontology clinical nurse specialists (CNS), and nurses with interest in geriatric practice who would provide oversight for the TWICE program. To develop and prioritize a work plan for staff education and quality improvement, NMHC nurses' attitudes, knowledge, and perceptions of providing care to older adults were identified. The Geriatric Institutional Assessment Profile (GIAP), developed by NICHE and made available to NICHE sites, was used to assess gerontological nursing practice around common geriatric syndromes (Abraham. Bottrell, Fulmer, & Mezey, 1999).

The GIAP results for NMHC indicated knowledge deficits for preventing skin breakdown, managing incontinence, and improving functional status for hospitalized elders. The results further indicated that nurses were frustrated with providing care for the "confused" patient. Palmateer and McCartney (1985) identified that staff nurses tend to use the term "confused" to describe patients with either dementia or delirium. Unfortunately, the lack of specificity in identifying the type of confusion leads to difficulty in identifying appropriate, effective nursing interventions. The nurses on the orthopedic unit often described feeling overwhelmed, ineffective, and physically and mentally exhausted after caring for extremely confused older adults with dementia, delirium, or both. Confusion was seen almost as a "normal consequence" of advanced age and a condition that is not amenable to nursing intervention.

The TWICE steering committee selected one of the NICHE practice models, the Geriatric Resource Nurse (GRN) model, to empower staff nurses to improve care for older adults and to address specifically the issue of confusion. The GRN model is a unit-based approach in which RNs who have agreed to become geriatric specialists serve as resources to other nurses and provide nursing care to complex elderly patients (NICHE Project Faculty, 1994). GRN development included nurses' attendance at geriatric conferences, and working with the CNS who used role modeling to teach geriatric-focused care.

The process for the GRN model started with the admitting staff nurse referring elders to the GRNs as a result of broad-based screening assessments based on NMHC's version of the acronym SPICES (i.e., safety, pain, incontinence, confusion, eating, and sleep impairment). The original SPICES acronym for the NICHE program (i.e., skin impairment, poor nutrition, incontinence, cognitive impairment, evidence of falls or functional decline, and sleep disturbance) (Fulmer, 1991) was modified to include a stronger focus on pain and safety. The GRNs and the CNS made rounds several times a week to elders referred to them to develop a care plan that addressed geriatric syndromes identified for the patient. "Rounds" included seeing the patient and conducting more thorough geriatric-focused assessments, especially using assessments geared toward identifying patients with delirium, dementia, or both.

The GRNs' and the CNS' most important assessment for confused patients was to identify a timeline for the confused state, which included determining whether the patient's confusion was an acute or chronic condition, which is more indicative of dementia. Through interviews with the patient and family and discussions with the primary physician, the patient's baseline level of cognition and functioning was clarified. The GRNs and the CNS then attempted to identify the approximate time the patient's functioning declined, as well as factors that may have precipitated or contributed to the decline. This information helped nurses target effective interventions for eliminating or decreasing the effect of those factors. The goal was to help the patient recover to a previous or an improved level of functioning.

UNIT-BASED APPROACH FOR MANAGING DELIRIUM

In 1999, the original TWICE unit was the orthopedic unit, a thirty-five-bed unit in which 40 to 60% of the unit's average daily census ($\overline{X}$ = 32) were patients 70 years of age or older. The primary diagnoses for elders were joint replacement and hip fracture repair. The orthopedic unit nurses selected the prevention and management of delirium as their first quality improvement focus based on the GIAP results and the iatrogenic nature and frequency of delirium for older orthopedic patients (Marcantonio, Flacker, Michaels, & Resnick, 2000).

Through a literature review, members of the TWICE steering committee identified a multi-intervention approach as important in preventing and managing delirium for patients with or without preexisting dementia. This approach includes staff education, standardized assessment of cognition, and identification of contributing factors with focused interventions that address those factors (Inouye et al., 1999; Marcantonio et al., 2001).

Staff Education

The need for staff education about delirium is well documented; physicians and nurses do not recognize that patients have delirium 33 to 66% of the time (Inouye et al., 1999). Many caregivers accept the onset of delirium or increase in its severity as inevitable for older adults, and differentiation between syndromes representing acute, potentially reversible states and those resulting from chronic conditions, with more permanent impairment, do not occur (Foreman, 1993). Health care professionals tend not to identify the fluctuating nature of delirium as a distinguishing feature; instead, this variable presentation tends to confound the ability to make a diagnosis (Inouye et al., 1999). More importantly, clinicians do not identify patient characteristics associated with the risk for delirium and, therefore, have no preventative care plan. Predictive studies identify age, dementia, bladder catheters, and physical restraints as predisposing factors for delirium (Inouye & Charpentier, 1996; Marcantonio, Goldman, Mangione, Ludwig, Muraca, & Haslauer, et al., 1994). Initially, the orthopedic unit staff did not clearly understand that patients with dementia commonly develop delirium with acute illness and hospitalization. If a patient was determined to have dementia, his or her declining cognition was viewed as a result of worsening dementia instead of acute illness. Thus, improving the patient's cognitive status was not always part of the care plan.

Without a focus on prevention and early recognition, patients often do not receive treatment until the delirium is severe. Interventions are delayed and not targeted toward preventing or managing the most salient causal factors (Eden & Foreman, 1996; Shedd, Kobokovich, & Slattery, 1995). Thus, the development of delirium with hospitalization is associated with mortality rates of 25 to 33% (Inouye et al., 1999). Based on a review of the literature, TWICE steering committee members deemed that education on assessments was the first priority. Prevention and treatment begins with accurately identifying elders at risk for delirium and those with the condition. Assessments should examine the same defining elements so delirium can be detected promptly and consistently (Foreman, 1993).

Staff education started with clarifying the concept of delirium, identifying the essential elements of the condition, and contrasting the condition with dementia. Members of the TWICE steering committee adopted the following definition: "Delirium is a transient state of cognitive impairment manifested by simultaneous disturbances of consciousness, attention, perception, memory, thinking, orientation, and psychomotor behavior that develop abruptly and fluctuate diurnally" (Foreman, 1993, p. 6). Staff development also included the use of the American Psychiatric Association DSM-IV (1994) criteria for diagnosing delirium, which includes: (1) disturbance of consciousness, (2) reduced ability to focus, sustain, or shift attention, (3) memory deficits, impairment of thinking, changes in perception with a tendency toward misperceptions, illusions and hallucinations, and language disturbances, and (4) acute onset with a relatively brief duration, with unpredictable fluctuations in alertness and cognition. A "roundtable" format was used to educate the orthopedic staff about assessing delirium; this format consisted of fifteen- to twenty-minute presentations of information, followed by twenty-five minutes of discussion, facilitated through the use of prepared questions. The goal was to involve staff and allow them to relate the new information to their own experiences and practices.

Standardized Cognitive Assessment Instruments

An assessment instrument, based on the essential features for delirium, was selected before completion of staff education. Standardized cognitive assessment tools are superior to relying on the individual clinician's assessment process for identifying delirium (Palmateer & McCartney, 1985). Three commonly used instruments in assessing cognition and delirium include the Mini-Mental Status Exam (MMSE) (Folstein, Folstein, & McHugh, 1975), the Confusion Assessment Method (CAM)

(Inouye, van Dyck, Alessi, Balkin, Siegal, & Horwitz, 1990), and the NEECHAM Acute Confusion Instrument (Neelon, Champagne, Carlson, & Funk, 1996).

The TWICE steering committee's requirements for choosing a standardized instrument included psychometric rigor, ease of administration and interpretation of results, ability to detect changes in clinical status, patient acceptability, and need for a screening and a monitoring instrument (Foreman, 1993). Based on these criteria, committee members selected the NEECHAM Acute Confusion Instrument, which is an observational assessment tool developed to be a rapid, unobtrusive assessment of cognitive and behavioral functions. The tool's main advantages are its sensitivity to the early onset of delirium, ability to be completed in five to ten minutes, and its ease of incorporation into daily practice with minimal instruction (Miller, Neelon, Champagne, Bailey, Ng'andu, & Belyea, et al., 1997). The NEECHAM instrument includes an assessment of the patient's cognitive processing ability, current behavior, and physiologic control to identify patients at risk and those currently suffering from delirium. Scores indicate normal functioning (27–30), risk for confusion (25–26), mild or early development of confusion (20–24), and moderate to severe confusion (0–19).

The TWICE steering committee members and the orthopedic nurses decided to initiate the NEECHAM instrument on admission for all older patients and then daily until discharge. The age of 70 was selected as the trigger, based on the average age of older patients admitted to the nursing units. Fifteen-minute between-shift education sessions were provided on the use of the NEECHAM instrument; examples of completed NEECHAM instrument were posted, and the CNS provided one-on-one support.

While the NEECHAM instrument has a high degree of clinical feasibility, the disadvantage is that it is not based on DSM delirium criteria, and specificity is an issue. Some authors advocate using a variety of measures for assessing delirium because no one instrument provides a complete assessment (Rapp, 2001). Several NICHE sites have adopted the CAM, which is an algorithm based on the DSM IIIR delirium criteria. The CAM is very effective for diagnosing delirium (Inouye et al., 1990; Marcantonio et al., 1994), but members of the TWICE steering committee determined it would not be effective to use in daily practice because the results are dichotomous (i.e., "yes," delirium is present, or "no," delirium is not present) and cannot be used for trending recovery. The CNSs at NMHC use the CAM to validate the presence of delirium when equivocal results occur with the NEECHAM. For example, a patient with a history of dementia may have an abnormal NEECHAM score because of dementia, but it is unclear if delirium is also present. The CAM includes questions to determine if there has been an acute change or worsening of confusion with a fluctuating course, inattention, disorganized thinking, or altered consciousness. These questions help determine whether or not delirium is present.

Because of validity and reliability issues of observational assessment tools, other NICHE sites advocate using the MMSE for assessing cognitive decline. However, while the MMSE does detect cognitive changes in patients with delirium, it does not differentiate delirium from dementia (Anthony, LeResche, Niaz, VonKorff, & Folstein, 1982). Prior to the initiation of the TWICE program, the NMHC nursing standards committee approved the use of the MMSE to assess cognitive decline in patients; however, few nurses used the instrument, and when they did, the reliability was poor. Nurses often lack knowledge in using formal mental status exams and view their use as an additional task requiring extra time (Palmateer & McCartney, 1985). Physicians have primarily designed mental status questionnaires; thus, these tools may fit better within medical versus nursing practice. Because the MMSE does have utility in assessing cognition, the gerontology CNS frequently uses the MMSE in assessing complex patients. For example, a patient may have a normal NEECHAM score but still seem to have some cognitive decline. Testing a patient's actual cognitive abilities may be the only way to determine if the patient is having difficulty. In the TWICE program, staff nurses and the CNS work as a team and use a variety of instruments to evaluate delirium and cognitive status in elders.

Identification of Contributing Factors and Focused Interventions

Lack of knowledge, as evidenced by the GIAP results, also existed for the orthopedic nurses regarding appropriate delirium interventions. This lack of knowledge is not unique to NMHC; many practicing nurses utilize a limited approach and primarily use restraints, sedation, and sitters. Interventions are not holistic and are generally aimed only at managing patient behavior and safety (Ludwick & O'Toole, 1996). Evidence from the patient's history, physical examination, or laboratory findings indicating a causal relationship between the presence of organic factors and delirium is an important part of the DSM-IV criteria. The etiology of delirium is generally multifactorial. Delirium can occur from acute illness, substance abuse, and sudden withdrawal from medications; interventions must be focused toward the etiology of the delirium. Intervening without knowledge of the specific cause(s) may result in ineffective and potentially dangerous care. For example, enhancing mobility for a patient with delirium is inappropriate if the etiology is from the combined effect of an electrolyte imbalance and the use of opioids and not immobility. The patient would not recover unless the right factors were addressed and the care individualized to the patient's needs.

Early nursing intervention studies on delirium examined psychosocial interventions such as providing reality orientation, family support, continuity of caregivers, and preoperative teaching, including anticipatory information about delirium (Cole, Primeau, & McCusker, 1996). Even though these studies were able to demonstrate improved outcomes, significant numbers of subjects still developed delirium or negative consequences. The same has been true for studies testing physiological delirium interventions, such as early surgical intervention for hip fracture repair or the use of preoperative thiamin (Day, Bayer, McMahon, Pathy, Spragg, & Rowlands, 1988; Gustafson et al., 1991).

Foreman (1993) concluded from these studies that single interventions focusing only on psychosocial or physiological factors are insufficient treatments. Holistic interventions that include both physiological and psychosocial actions are more effective in a structured care process. Another conclusion can also be drawn: The majority of these studies did not determine the actual etiology of delirium in their study population prior to designing the intervention; thus, it is possible these interventions were not focused or directed at the underlying causal factors, which limited the success of the intervention. There may be potential value for using algorithms, protocols, or guidelines for assisting caregivers in identifying the multiple causal factors present for their patients and in matching appropriate interventions.

The delirium protocol developed for NICHE (Foreman, Mion, Tryostad, & Fletcher, 1999) was selected as the basis for the orthopedic quality improvement project, because it was designed for use in a wide variety of elderly patient populations. The protocol was modified to include the best features from other delirium standards (Foreman, 1984; American Psychiatric Association, 1999). The focus for the protocol was the management of delirium, and the expected outcome was the reduction of the severity and length of the delirium for patients with or without preexisting dementia. The roundtable format was used again to teach pharmacologic and non-pharmacologic methods for preventing and managing delirium, and between-shift training sessions were used to highlight the new delirium protocol.

Outcome Measures

The primary patient focus for the initial outcomes included orthopedic patients who were at least 70 years of age and had normal or at-risk NEECHAM scores on admission. This population included patients who had either normal cognition or a mild form of dementia prior to hospitalization. The goal for this population was to reduce the incidence of delirium, decrease the number of days or severity of the delirium, and achieve a normal NEECHAM score prior to discharge. Because these patients did not have delirium on admission, the nursing staff had opportunities to prevent its occurrence because of the iatrogenic nature of the condition. Orthopedic patients admitted with abnormal NEECHAM scores were identified as a different population in which dementia was a common comorbidity. These patients were included in the measure of prevalence. The goal for this population was to reduce the number of days or severity of the delirium and to improve the discharge NEE-CHAM score. In addition, even though the orthopedic unit used restraints as a last resort, the staff wanted to decrease the average time a confused patient was restrained. The TWICE operational definitions for the selected outcomes are found in Table 9.1.

From baseline to 2000, the majority of orthopedic patients admitted with abnormal NEECHAM scores and those developing delirium during hospitalization were female and 80 years of age or older (see Table 9.2, A & B). A high percentage of patients admitted with abnormal NEECHAM scores (71–89%; see Table 9.2A) had histories of dementia versus those who developed delirium with hospitalization (8–13%; see Table 9.2B). Additionally, comparison of the lowest NEECHAM scores (i.e., severity of delirium) during hospitalization ($\overline{X}$ = 16.53 / SD 6.49 – 18.23 / SD 6.11) and the discharge NEECHAM scores ($\overline{X}$ = 20 / SD 6.85 – 22 / SD 6.18) demonstrates a difference in scores that gives some support to the belief that many of the orthopedic patients with abnormal NEECHAM

TABLE 9.1   Operational Definitions for Delirium Outcomes on the Orthopedic Unit

Outcomes	Measurement
Incidence of delirium: not present on admission, but occurring during hospitalization	Admission NEECHAM score > 24 with at least one score < 25 while hospitalized
Prevalence of confusion (either delirium or dementia, or both): present on admission	Admission NEECHAM score < 25 on admission
Severity of delirium	Lowest NEECHAM score obtained while hospitalized
Severity of delirium at discharge	NEECHAM score on day of discharge from the hospital
Days of delirium	Number of hospital days with NEECHAM scores < 25
Average time in restraints	Total hours restrained

scores on admission had delirium (see Table 9.3A). Specifically, as these patients recovered, their NEECHAM scores increased, indicating cognitive improvements, even for those patients with a preexisting dementia.

The incidence of delirium for all orthopedic patients with normal or at-risk NEECHAM scores on admission was 20% ($n = 199$) at baseline, and at the end of 1999, the overall incidence rate was 11.7% ($n = 881$) for the year (see Table 9.2B). The results demonstrated a steady decline every month and reached the lowest level of 4.8% ($n = 63$) in December 1999. No change occurred with the severity or the number of days of delirium for this population (see Table 9.3A). However, delirium severity and the discharge NEECHAM scores did improve slightly for patients admitted with abnormal NEECHAM scores (Lowest NEECHAM score:

TABLE 9.2   Demographics: Orthopedic Elders 70 Years and Older

A. Confused on Admission to the Hospital: Prevalence*

Year sample	Number and % of confused elders	Age (mean/SD) of confused elders	% Female confused elders	% Confused elders with dementia
Baseline 6/99–8/99 $n = 199$	$f = 44$ 22%	$\overline{X} = 80.73$ $SD = 6.52$	54	88.64
1999 $n = 881$	$f = 197$ 22.4%	$\overline{X} = 82.24$ $SD = 6.91$	56.2	63.8
2000 $n = 693$	$f = 150$ 21.6%	$\overline{X} = 82.85$ $SD = 9.30$	66.7	70.9

*Prevalence: confused on admission due to delirium, dementia, or both delirium and dementia.

B. Elders Developing Delirium with Hospitalization: Incidence**

Year sample	Number and % elders with delirium	Age (mean/SD) of confused elders	% Female confused elders	% Elders with delirium and dementia
Baseline 6/99–8/99 $n = 199$	$f = 40$ 20%	$\overline{X} = 80.73$ $SD = 6.52$	66.7	12.8
1999 $n = 881$	$f = 81$ 11.7%	$\overline{X} = 82.24$ $SD = 6.91$	67.1	12.3
2000 $n = 693$	$f = 91$ 12.9%	$\overline{X} = 82.85$ $SD = 9.30$	57.3	7.7

**Incidence: the development of delirium during hospitalization.

TABLE 9.3 Outcomes: Orthopedic Patients 70 Years and Older

A. Confused on Admission: Prevalence*

Year sample	Days of confusion (mean/SD)	Severity: lowest NEECHAM (mean/SD)	Discharge NEECHAM (mean/SD)	Length of stay (mean/SD)
Baseline 6/99–7/99 n = 199	$\overline{X}$ = 3.9 SD = 2.17	$\overline{X}$ = 16.55 SD = 6.79	$\overline{X}$ = 20 SD = 6.85	$\overline{X}$ = 4.6 SD = 3.59
1999 n = 881	$\overline{X}$ = 3.7 SD = 2.29	$\overline{X}$ = 16.53 SD = 6.49	$\overline{X}$ = 21 SD = 6.73	$\overline{X}$ = 4.5 SD = 2.84
2000 n = 693	$\overline{X}$ = 3.6 SD = 2.02	$\overline{X}$ = 18.23 SD = 6.11	$\overline{X}$ = 22 SD= 6.18	$\overline{X}$ = 4.4 SD = 2.62

*Prevalence: confused on admission due to delirium, dementia, or both delirium and dementia.

B. Elders Developing Delirium with Hospitalization: Incidence**

Year sample	Days of delirium (mean/SD)	Severity: lowest NEECHAM (mean/SD)	Discharge NEECHAM (mean/SD)	Length of stay (mean/SD)
Baseline 6/99–8/99 n = 199	$\overline{X}$ = 1.77 SD = .95	$\overline{X}$ = 21.21 SD = 3.38	$\overline{X}$ = 26.5 SD = 3.16	$\overline{X}$ = 4.5 SD = 1.95
1999 n = 881	$\overline{X}$ = 1.66 SD = .89	$\overline{X}$ = 21.65 SD = 3.07	$\overline{X}$ = 26.9 SD = 2.96	$\overline{X}$ = 4.8 SD = 2.19
2000 n = 693	$\overline{X}$ = 2.75 SD = 3.12	$\overline{X}$ = 21.59 SD = 4.85	$\overline{X}$ = 26.6 SD = 3.74	$\overline{X}$ = 6.15 SD = 4.06

**Incidence: the development of delirium during hospitalization.

$\overline{X}$ = 16.55 to 18.23; Discharge NEECHAM score: $\overline{X}$ = 20 to 22) (see Table 9.3B). Also, the average time all confused patients were restrained decreased from two days to 22 hours.

While the incidence rate of 4.8% was not sustained, the rate in 2000 did not return to baseline (see Table 9.2B). The TWICE steering committee narrowed the focus of the project in 2001 to elderly patients admitted with hip fractures, since 40% of patients who developed delirium in 1999 and 2000 were admitted with this diagnosis. Through retrospective chart reviews, contributing factors for delirium were identified and included the prolonged use of bladder catheters, poor nutrition, dehydration, and inadequate pain management. Improvement initiatives promoted the discontinuation of bladder catheters by the second postoperative day, standardizing pain management and adding a pain management CNS to the interdisciplinary team, early referral to nutrition services and use of nutritional supplements for patients at high risk for malnutrition, and ensuring adequate hydration. The incidence of delirium for older adults with hip fractures did demonstrate a decline from 21.2% ($n = 146$) in 1999 to 18% ($n = 172$) in 2000 and 12.8 to 12.9% ($n = 211$ and $n = 202$) in 2001 and 2002. Overall, the TWICE program at the unit level has shown to be effective in changing practice.

ORGANIZATION-BASED APPROACH
FOR MANAGING DELIRIUM

There were several factors in 2002 that led NMHC to progress from a unit-based approach to an organizational approach for addressing delirium. From the beginning of the TWICE program, a major goal was to address the needs of older adults at an organizational level. The TWICE steering committee members recognized that nursing units are not closed systems. Specifically, nurses floating from other units do not necessarily know gerontological principles. Also, a variety of physicians care for elders, and some physicians are unaware of TWICE and do not place the same importance on the TWICE nurses' recommendations. Staff turnover, even when minimal, must be addressed through ongoing TWICE orientation.

The TWICE steering committee members recommended an indirect method to diffuse information, to increase awareness of geriatric issues, and to change clinical processes to be more supportive of older adults by having GRNs serve on task teams or committees to address organizational issues. Outcomes of this approach have included the development of nursing education programs for skin assessment and integration of geriatric assessment tools, such as the Braden scale (Bergstrom, Braden, Laguzza, & Homan, 1987) for determining risk for skin breakdown, the Blaylock scale (Blaylock & Cason, 1992) for identifying discharge-planning needs, and the Hendrich Fall Risk Assessment (Hendrich, 1996), into the nursing admission form and daily flow sheets.

NMHC selected delirium prevention as one of five organizational safety initiatives due to its broad implications. Specifically, safety issues associated with delirium include increased falls and injuries, adverse drug events, restraints, and the need for sitters to observe and protect patients with delirium. NMHC is promoting Inouye's view that delirium provides "a window to hospital care" regarding the overall quality of care for the geriatric population (Inouye et al., 1999). The opportunity to change iatrogenic practices associated with delirium on a broader scale, such as inappropriate use of psychoactive medications, poor nutritional management, prolonged immobilization, prevention of sleep, and the overuse of bladder catheters and restraints, increases the likelihood of reducing the incidence of delirium as well as improving the overall care for elders throughout the organization. An interdisciplinary delirium task team was established to capitalize on the experience from the orthopedic unit and to apply that knowledge to change other systems in the organization.

The framework for the delirium safety initiative included recommendations made by Inouye et al. (1999), the NICHE organizational model to improve detection and management of delirium, and interventions implemented as part of NMHC's unit-based model. The focus areas include ensuring cognitive assessment for all elders, strategies to change practice patterns, clinical guidelines, individualized nursing interventions, enhanced geriatric expertise at the bedside, and staff education.

Cognitive Assessment of All Older Patients

Initially, the NEECHAM instrument was utilized only on the orthopedic unit and was used for patients aged 70 years or older. Beginning March 2003, use of the NEECHAM was extended to all adult medical/surgical units at NMHC and was changed to be used for patients 75 years or older. The age was increased, based on the average age of patients with delirium on the orthopedic unit (see Tables 9.2A and 9.2B). Nursing staff on some of the medical/surgical units had difficulty consistently completing the NEECHAM on admission because they were not involved in the initial TWICE program and struggled with the instrument's value when prioritizing their daily work. Education regarding the benefit of standardized assessment instruments is important in ensuring compliance. Availability of the instrument was problematic, which was solved by having the tool placed on the computer and with the admission paperwork.

Strategies to Change Practice Patterns

A process was initiated for reviewing preprinted orders for medications known to cause delirium in elders and that require age-specific dosing parameters. Diphenhydramine, propoxyphene, meperidine, triazolam, and hydroxyzine are key medications being removed from the orders (Beers, 1997). The pharmacy has installed a new system that has the capability of alerting pharmacists of medication issues. The alert-system rules that identify inappropriate medications, dosages, and drug combinations that have high likelihoods for causing adverse drug reactions in older patients are being established.

Clinicians are being asked to evaluate the need for urinary catheters and to promote their early removal. Preprinted surgical orders include automatic orders to discontinue catheters. Urinary catheters are often continued because of the patient's immobility, fatigue, staff convenience, and physician unawareness of the catheter's presence (Saint, Lipsky, & Gould, 2002). Staff and physician education is an important intervention for appropriate catheter use.

Clinical Guidelines

The original TWICE protocol addressed delirium management and has evolved to include prevention (included in the appendix to this chapter). A predictive delirium model based on the interrelationship between the patient's baseline vulnerability and contributing factors serves as the framework for assessment and intervention (Inouye & Charpentier, 1996; Lipowski, 1990). Three categories of factors are included in the protocol: predisposing, precipitating, and facilitating. Predisposing factors are conditions that increase the likelihood a person will develop delirium. A screening section has been added to the nursing admission form and includes the following predisposing factors: age of 75 or older; substance abuse; sensory impairment; and history of acute confusion, depression, stroke, dementia, or other types of brain injuries. Positive answers to the screen trigger the use of the NEECHAM assessment instrument and the delirium protocol.

Precipitating factors are organic causes considered necessary for delirium to occur and include systemic disease, medication effects, and withdrawal from substances. Facilitating factors are viewed as common contributing factors that are neither necessary nor sufficient for directly causing delirium; rather, they increase the severity and length of the delirium. However, there is some debate that facilitating factors may be sufficient to cause delirium for patients with dementia. Facilitating factors include unfamiliar environments, isolation, emotional stress, and pain (Kozak-Campbell & Hughes, 1996; Lipowski, 1990). The protocol is written to help nurses determine appropriate interventions based on factors in the patient's presentation.

Individualized Delirium Interventions

Several interventions for patients with delirium are individualized and based on facilitating factors that may exist. Behavioral changes are assessed with respect to patient needs for pain control, ambulation, opportunities for elimination, food, water, and reassurance and presence (Kolanowski, 1999). These interventions are especially important for patients with dementia in order to prevent delirium from occurring. Patients with dementia have limited cognitive reserves to combat the stress associated with illness; meeting those patients' basic needs and managing the environment are important in preventing additional stress. A "busy box" is a new intervention that may have potential for reducing agitation from inactivity. The "busy box" items, such as pictures for reminiscing, may distract the confused patient from pulling out tubes or getting up without assistance. Medications to manage delirium are used as a last resort and are targeted toward psychotic symptoms such as hallucinations and delusions.

An intervention designed to prevent falls is the bed-alarm (AGS Panel on Falls in Older Persons, 2001), which includes features for controlling the volume, delay, and type of alarm sound. A taped message from the patient's family or nursing staff can help keep the patient from getting up on his or her own. For confused patients whose first language is not English or who are fearful of nursing staff, having a family member's or a friend's recorded voice is especially useful.

A teaching sheet on delirium is available for nurses to use as an intervention to address families' fears and anxieties. The content includes a description of delirium, potential causes, the expected course and duration, comfort and safety needs, and treatments. Helping the family understand differences among delirium and dementia and the combination of both conditions is an important aspect of family education.

Enhanced Geriatric Expertise at the Bedside

Nurses need resources for expert consultation for managing complex geriatric care. The NICHE organizational model for improving management of delirium uses the expertise of a gerontology CNS for: (1) support in assessing cognition, (2) assistance in distinguishing delirium from dementia and depression, (3) accurate communication with physicians, (4) identification of factors contributing to delirium, (5) application of independent, collaborative, and delegated interventions for preventing and managing delirium, and (6) documenting findings in the patient record (NICHE Project Faculty, 1994). The unit-based approach depends on collaboration between GRNs and CNSs, while the organizational approach includes a hospital-wide referral process for CNS consultation because most areas do not have GRNs. NMHC has medical-surgical gerontology and psychiatric CNSs who respond to referrals for geriatric patients diagnosed with delirium. A major focus of the CNS is to help staff implement and individualize the delirium protocol to each patient and ensure interdisciplinary collaboration.

Staff Education

Organizational education initiatives for managing and preventing delirium are being developed through collaboration among the TWICE steering committee, CNSs, and the education department. A variety of organizational education initiatives include a competency on the NEE-CHAM instrument to increase the number of geriatric-certified nurses, inclusion of "delirium" as a topic at the annual medical-surgical conference, and the new RN graduate program.

Several innovative approaches to staff education have been initiated. The gerontology CNS created a jigsaw "delirium puzzle" in which staff uses pieces describing contributing factors to complete the puzzle. A video and facilitator's training guide, "Clinical Judgment and Advocacy for the Older Hospitalized Patient," tells the story of a hospitalized elder who develops delirium; it is used at interdisciplinary forums. The video offers opportunities to discuss many issues with clinicians regarding advocacy for older patients, accountabilities, and the experiences of family members.

CONCLUSION

Delirium prevention is a necessary part of acute care. Building on research and best practice models like NICHE, NMHC's unit-based approach was instrumental in decreasing the incidence of delirium. Due to this success, the hospital selected the reduction of delirium as an organizational safety initiative. Support was given to Inouye, Schlesinger, and Lydon's (1999) idea to use the incidence of delirium as a "window to hospital care" for geriatric patients. The relationship of delirium and the overall quality of geriatric care is being recognized.

The key elements of an organizational approach in reducing delirium include: cognitive assessment for elders, strategies to change practice patterns, a delirium protocol that includes prevention, individualized nursing interventions focused on facilitating factors, availability of CNS consultation throughout the institution, and staff education. NMHC is in the beginning phases of implementing an organizational approach, and outcomes are too early to report; however, we are committed to working toward quality geriatric care and reducing the incidence of delirium.

REFERENCES

References to TWICE Protocol

American Journal of Psychiatry (1999). Practice guideline for the treatment of patients with delirium. May; 156 (5 Suppl), 1–20.

Inouye, S. K., & Charpentier, P. A. (1996). Precipitating factors for delirium in hospitalized elderly persons: Predictive model and interrelationship with baseline vulnerability. The Journal of the American Medical Association, 275 (11), 852–857.

Marcantonio, E. R., Flacker, J. M., Wright, J., & Resnick, N. M. (2001). Reducing delirium after hip fracture: A randomized trial. Journal of the American Geriatrics Society, 49, 516–522.

Neelon, V. J., Champagne, M. T., Carson, J. R., & Funk, S. G. (1996). The NEECHAM confusion scale: Construction, validation, and clinical testing. Nursing Research, 45 (6), 324–330.

REFERENCES

Abraham, I., Bottrell, M., Dash, K., Fulmer, T., Mezey, M., & O'Donnell, L., et al. (1999). Profiling care and benchmarking best practice in care of hospitalized elderly. *Nursing Clinics of North America, 34*(2), 239–253.

AGS (American Geriatric Society Panel on Falls in Older Persons) (2001). Guideline for the prevention of falls in older persons. *American Geriatrics Society, 49*(5), 664–672.

American Psychiatric Association (1994). *Diagnostic and statistical manual of mental disorders.* (4th ed.), Washington, DC: APA.

American Psychiatric Association (1999). Practice guideline for the treatment of patients with delirium. *American Journal of Psychiatry, 156S, 1–20.

Anthony, J., LeResche, L., Niaz, U., Von Korff, M., & Folstein, M. (1982). Limits of the Mini-Mental State' as a screening test for dementia and delirium among hospital patients. *Psychological Medicine, 12*(2), 397–408.

Beers, M. (1997). Explicit criteria for determining potentially inappropriate medication use by the elderly. *Archives of Internal Medicine, 157*(14), 1531–1536.

Bergstrom, N., Braden, B., Laguzza, A., & Homan, Z. (1987). The Braden Scale for predicting pressure sore risk. *Nursing Research, 36*(4), 205–210.

Blaylock, A. & Cason, C. (1992). Discharge planning: Predicting patients' needs. *Journal of Gerontological Nursing, 18*(7), 5–10.

Cole, M., Primeau, F., & McCusker, J. (1996). Effectiveness of interventions to prevent delirium in hospitalized patients: a systematic review. *Canadian Medical Association Journal, 155*(9), 1263–1268.

Day, J., Bayer, A. McMahon, M., Pathy, M., Spragg, B, & Rowlands, D. (1988). Thiamin status, vitamin supplements and postoperative confusion. *Age and Ageing, 17*(1), 29–34.

Eden, B. M., & Foreman, M. D. (1996). Problems associated with underrecognition of delirium in critical care: A case study. *Heart and Lung, 25*(5), 388–400.

Folstein, M., Folstein, S. & McHugh, P. (1975). "Mini-Mental State" a practical method for grading the cognitive state of patients for the clinician. *Journal of Psychiatric Research, 12*(3), 189–198.

Foreman, M. (1984). Acute confusional states in the elderly: An algorithm. *Dimensions of Critical Care Nursing, 3*(4), 207–215.

Foreman, M. (1993). Acute confusion in the elderly. *Annual Review of Nursing Research, 11*, 3–30.

Foreman, M., Mion, L., Tryostad, L., & Fletcher, K. (1999). Standard of practice protocol: Acute confusion/delirium. *Geriatric Nursing, 20*(3), 147–152.

Fulmer, T. (1991). The geriatric nurse specialist role: A new model. *Nursing Management, 22*(3), 91–93.

Gustafson, Y., Brannstrom, B., Berggren, D., Ragnarsson, J., Sigaard, J., & Bucht, G., et al. (1991). A geriatric-anesthesiologic program to reduce acute confusional states in the elderly patients treated for femoral neck fractures. *Journal of the American Geriatrics Society, 39*(7), 655–662.

Hendrich, A. (1996). *Falls, immobility, and restraints: A resource manual.* St. Louis: Mosby.

Inouye, S., van Dyck, C., Alessi, C., Balkin, S., Siegal, A., & Horwitz, R., et al. (1990). Clarifying confusion: The confusion assessment method a new method for detection of delirium. *Annals of Internal Medicine, 113*(12), 941–948.

Inouye, S., & Charpentier, P. (1996). Precipitating factors for delirium in hospitalized elderly persons: Predictive model and interrelationship with baseline vulnerability. *Journal of the American Medical Association, 275*(11), 852–857.

Inouye, S., Bogardus, S., Charpentier, P., Leo-summers, L., Acampora, D., & Holford, T., et al. (1999). A multicomponent intervention to prevent delirium in hospitalized older patients. *New England Journal of Medicine, 340*(9), 669–676.

Inouye, S., Schlesinger, M., & Lydon, T. (1999). Delirium: A symptom of how hospital care is failing older persons and a window to improve quality of hospital care. *The American Journal of Medicine, 106*(5), 565–573.

Kirkland, L. (1995). Delirium, DRGs, and documentation. *Archives of Internal Medicine, 155*(21), 2355.

Kolanowski, A. (1999). An overview of the need-driven dementia-compromised behavior model. *Journal of Gerontological Nursing, 25*(9), 7–9.

Kozak-Campbell, C., & Hughes, A. (1996). The use of functional consequences theory in acutely confused hospitalized elderly. *Journal of Gerontological Nursing, 22*(1), 27–36.

Lipowski, Z. (1990). *Delirium: Acute confusional states.* New York: Oxford University Press.

Ludwick, R., & O'Toole, A. (1996). The confused patient: nurses' knowledge and interventions. *Journal of Gerontological Nursing, 22*(1), 44–49.

Marcantonio, E., Goldman, L., Mangione, C., Ludwig, L., Muraca, B., & Haslauer, C., et al. (1994). A clinical prediction rule for delirium after elective noncardiac surgery. *Journal of the American Medical Association, 271*(2), 134–139.

Marcantonio, E., Flacker, J., Michaels, M., & Resnick, N. (2000). Delirium is independently associated with poor functional recovery after hip fracture. *Journal of the American Geriatrics Society, 48*(6), 618–624.

Marcantonio, E., Flacker, J., Wright, J., & Resnick, N. (2001). Reducing delirium after hip fracture: A randomized trial. *Journal of the American Geriatrics Society, 49*(5), 516–522.

Miller, J., Neelon, V., Champagne, M., Bailey, D., Ng'andu, N., & Belyea, M., et al. (1997). The assessment of acute confusion as part of nursing care. *Applied Nursing Research, 10*(3), 143–151.

Neelon, V., Champagne, M., Carlson, J. & Funk, S. (1996). The NEECHAM confusion scale: Construction, validation, and clinical testing. *Nursing Research, 45*(6), 324–330.

NICHE Project Faculty (1994). Geriatric models of care: Which one's right for your institution? Nurses Improving Care to Hospitalized Elders (NICHE) Project. *American Journal of Nursing, 17*(7), 222–227.

Palmateer, L., & McCartney, J. (1985). Do nurses know when patients have cognitive deficits? *Journal of Gerontological Nursing, 11*(2), 6–16.

Rapp, C. (2001). Acute confusion/delirium protocol. *Journal of Gerontological Nursing, 27*(4), 21–33.

Saint, S., Lipsky, B., & Gould, S. (2002). Indwelling urinary catheters: A one-point restraint? *Annals of Internal Medicine, 137*(2), 125–127.

Shedd, P. P., Kobokovich, L. J., & Slattery, M. J. (1995). Confused patients in the acute care setting: Prevalence, interventions, and outcomes. *Journal of Gerontological Nursing, 21*(4), 5–12.

Sparks, M. (2001). Assessment and management of Alzheimer's disease. *Medscape Nursing, 1*(2), Available from www.medscape.com/Medscape/Nurses/journal/2001/v01.n02/ mns0817.03.spar/mns0817.03spar01.html

The TWICE Protocol Delirium Prevention and Management

PROTOCOL

CONFUSION, ACUTE (DELIRIUM): PREVENTION AND MANAGEMENT

Supersedes: Confusion Protocol	Reviewed by: Delirium Task Team | Patient Care Practice | & Outcome | Date:	Approved: _____	Effective Date: 3/03

Personnel: RN's, LPN's, MHA's and NA's

Outcome goals:

1. Prevent delirium from occurring with hospitalization.

2. Decrease the severity and duration of delirium for patients who develop the syndrome.

Supportive Data: Theoretical framework adopted from Dr. Sharon Inouye's **Predictive Model** based on the interrelationship between the patient's baseline vulnerability and with other contributing factors.

1. Delirium is primarily multifactorial and identification of a single cause frequently leads to an incomplete plan of care. Three types of factors (i.e., predisposing, precipitating, and facilitating) usually contribute to the development, severity, and duration of delirium (see the table below).

2. The greater the number of predisposing factors, indicating higher patient vulnerability at baseline, the fewer precipitating and facilitating factors are needed to cause an episode of delirium.

3. The fewer predisposing factors, indicating less patient vulnerability at baseline, the greater number of precipitating and facilitating factors that are needed to cause an episode of delirium.

Predisposing Factors	Precipitating Factors	Facilitating Factors
(Vulnerability factors that increase a patient's risk or likelihood of developing delirium)	*(Physiological factors that are known to directly contribute to the development of delirium)*	*(Environmental, psychosocial, comfort, and functional issues that when present facilitate the onset, increase the severity or duration of delirium, but are generally not directly contributory without other physiological factors)*
Advanced age ≥75	Medications with CNS effects: sedatives, hypnotics, opioids, NSAIDS, Histamine-2 Receptor Antagonists, Digoxin	Immobility
Sensory impairment	Fluid & electrolyte imbalances	Elimination
History of acute confusion	Metabolic changes (e.g., hypoxia, hyper/hypo glycemia, decreased Hgb)	Changes in the environment
Pre-existing cognitive impairment — dementia — Parkinson's Disease — stroke — brain injury	Nutritional deficiencies	Pain and discomfort
Depression	Trauma	Anxiety
Substance abuse	Neurological event	Insufficient lighting
Cardiac disease & multiple chronic illnesses	Infections (e.g., pneumonia, UTI's)	Restraints
Functional impairment		Other tethering devices that tend to decrease the patient's mobility (e.g., IV, O2, cannula, Foley catheter, telemetry)
Fall in last 30 days		
At risk NEECHAM score of 25 or 26 or Blaylock score of ≥14		

(continued)

Protocol: Confusion, Acute (Delirium): Prevention and Management (continued)

Interventional goals:

1. Identify all contributing factors that may be present: predisposing, precipitating and facilitating factors. Work to eliminate or modify the effects of identified contributing factors

I. Prevention of Delirium: Starts with Identifying Patients at Risk		Support Functional Status: Prevent Decline
Assessments	Referrals	Interventions
Predisposing factors: Database: Age, Acute Confusion Risk section, Blaylock score greater or equal to 14		1. For patients greater or equal to age 75 or at high risk for cognitive impairment initiate the NEECHAM Acute Confusion Instrument (from SOE). 2. Confer with family/facility regarding baseline cognitive and functional (ADL's) levels, previous episodes of acute confusion, and potential causes and treatments.
Predisposing Factors: Database: Substance abuse and Alcohol Withdrawal.	Consider Psych CNS, Social Service	1. CIWA initiation and Alcohol Withdrawal Protocol.
Home Medications: Review Medication Verification Form. New Medications: Assess the patient's response (intended versus adverse).	Consider Pharmacist drug review if patient is at high risk for delirium or is on greater than or equal to 9 medications and is greater or equal to age 75.	1. Avoid abrupt cessation of home medications; work with physician & pharmacist to simplify medication regimen. 2. Patients greater or equal to age 75 avoid administration of new medications from the following drug classes when possible: anticholinergics (Benadryl, Vistaril), histamine-2 receptor blockers, sedative/hypnotics, benzodiazepines (e.g., Xanax, Valium, Ativan), antiemetics, antispasmodics.

Assessments	Referrals	Interventions
Nutrition: Database: Nutrition risk assessment and feeding needs. **Appetite and ability to eat:** Assess for nausea and vomiting, amount eaten, chewing and swallowing with each meal. **I & O:** Accurate	On admission, Dietitian Referral if: 1) triggered on database 2) Braden score less than 13 3) Blaylock greater or equal to 14 During hospitalization refer for poor intake, nutritional teaching, and diet planning.	1. Supplements. 2. Assist with tray setup/ feeding. Make sure patient has dentures in at mealtime, up in chair to to eat. 3. Provide culturally appropriate meals.
Cognitive/Perceptual: NEECHAM assessment daily and prn with suspected cognitive changes.	Consider Gerontology CNS referral for at risk scores (abnormal NEECHAM scores less than 25).	1. Make sure patient wears glasses & hearing aids. 2. Adequate lighting in room, use night-light. 3. Reality cues: calendar, clocks. 4. Reality reorientation incorporated in normal care activities (e.g., Good morning, it is Monday and here is your breakfast). 5. Avoid frequent room changes. 6. Shades up during day and closed during night. 7. Provide interpreters to patients who do not speak English. 8. Encourage families to bring in familiar items (e.g., pillows, pictures, blanket).

(continued)

Protocol: Confusion, Acute (Delirium): Prevention and Management (continued)

Assessments	Referrals	Interventions
Pain management: Pain ratings above 4, the patient's pain goal, and/or prevents function. *(Remember increased agitation may indicate poor pain control).*	Pain CNS for unmanageable pain or for complex pain management problems.	1. Provide adequate pain management. Use combination of opioids, acetaminophen, and non-pharmacologic interventions. 2. Avoid use of Demerol, Darvocet, Nubain, or Talwin. 3. For older patients and those at risk for confusion, substitute Dilaudid for morphine. Remember, start low, go slow. 4. Consider round-the-clock acetaminophen (watch total dose less than 4,000 mg/24 hours).
Elimination: **Database:** Last BM prior to admission and bowel pattern, Voiding issues CCFS: BMs during hospitalization, I & O.		1. Remove indwelling urine catheter ASAP. 2. Toilet every two hours. 3. Provide fluids. 4. Bowel program (recommend Senokot S for patients on opioids).
Immobility: **Database:** Blaylock assessment	PT (need MD order)	1. Chair for every meal. 2. Walk in halls. 3. Passive ROM. 4. Turn every two hours.
Safety: **Database:** Fall Score		1. Adequate lighting in room. 2. Fall protocol.
Stress/Coping: **Database:** Assess spiritual, cultural, and emotional needs.	Chaplain	1. Incorporate cultural and spiritual needs into the patient's plan of care. 2. Encourage families to be part of caregiving if it helps to provide a calming, routine environment. 3. Educate families about the risk for Delirium and ways they can help to prevent the condition. 4. Use consistent caregivers.

Assessments	Referrals	Interventions
Physiological Stability *(NEECHAM score of 25–26 at risk score most often due to Physiological control page 4)*		1. Monitor lab values: Blood chemistries specifically sodium, potassium, glucose, calcium, BUN, creatinine, and CBC. 2. Monitor UA/UC. 3. Monitor chest x-ray, ECG, oxygen saturations, keeping O2 levels greater than 92%. 4. Monitor drug levels or screens. 5. Monitor vital signs. 6. Observe for signs of infection *(mouth, teeth, and feet most overlooked source of infection).* 7. Address changes in physiological stability: reporting to the physician and implementing corrective interventions *(immediate corrections may prevent delirium).*

(continued)

Protocol: Confusion, Acute (Delirium): Prevention and Management (continued)

Management of Delirium		Improve Functional Status:
ALL OF THE ABOVE ASSESSMENTS, REFERRALS & INTERVENTIONS PLUS THE FOLLOWING:		
Assessments	Referrals	Interventions
Nutrition risk:	Dietitian referral	1. Provide fluids minimum of 1500 cc/24 hour (30 ml/kg) unless cardiac/renal disease. 2. Determine source of dehydration (e.g. medications, decreased fluid intake, infection).
Cognitive/Perceptual	OT referral CNS referral	1. Validate patient's feelings. Do not confront their reality; gentle validation of reality. 2. Remove meaningless and unnecessary stimuli. 3. Use a need driven approach to address and manage behavior: Is the patient having pain, hungry, needing to go to the bathroom, frightened, lonely, cold, hot, tired, wanting to get out of bed etc.? 4. When a patient is exhibiting psychotic symptoms (hallucinations or paranoia) which cause patient distress or impairs functional capacity, contact physician and discuss low dose antipsychotic. 5. Ativan is not recommended for any of the symptoms listed in number 4. 6. Patient/Family education about delirium (obtain on SOE).
Safety		1. Posey sitter II, falling star sign. 2. Safety policy/procedure initiated. 3. Room near the desk. 4. Bed check.

Assessments	Referrals	Interventions
Post-procedure		1. Limit pre-procedural sedation if patient at high risk for post procedural confusion, give lowest dose of sedation medications. 2. Assess for effects of pre-, peri- and post-procedure medications and interactions.
Discharge planning needs: Blaylock score greater than 9	Social Service and Home Health referral (need MD order)	1. Family Education/ instruction concerning safety needs, medications, return appointments, activity, and diet.

References

Abraham, I., Bottrell, M.M., Fulmer, T., & Mezey, M.D. (1999). Geriatric Nursing Protocols for Best Practice, New York: Springer.

American Journal of Psychiatry (1999). Practice guideline for the treatment of patients with delirium. May; 156 (5 Suppl), 1–20.

Inouye, S.K., & Charpentier, P.A. (1996). Precipitating factors for delirium in hospitalized elderly persons: Predictive model and interrelationship with baseline vulnerability. The Journal of the American Medical Association, 275 (11), 852–857.

Marcantonio, E.R., Flacker, J.M., Wright, J., & Resnick, N.M. (2001). Reducing delirium after hip fracture: A randomized trial. *Journal of the American Geriatrics Society,* 49, 516–522.

Neelon, V.J., Champagne, M.T., Carson, J.R., & Funk, S.G. (1996). The NEECHAM confusion scale: Construction, validation, and clinical testing. *Nursing Research,* 45 (6), 324–330.

CHAPTER TEN

Care of the Patient with Dementia in the Acute Care Setting

The Role of the ACE Unit

Cheryl A. Lehman, Susan Tyler, and Luis Felipe Amador

The older adult faces many risks during hospitalization for an acute illness. An unfamiliar setting, strange faces and routines, multiple tests and procedures, as well as decreased mobility and poor nutritional intake can all lead to complications throughout the hospitalization. These complications can include deconditioning, falls, delirium and agitation, incontinence, and infection. The challenge in acute care for older adults is to treat the acute illness while preventing complications, maintaining function and self care abilities, and planning for a successful discharge to the least restrictive environment.

The patient with dementia presents added challenges to the acute care provider. Ethical, safety, and psychosocial issues directly related to the dementia must be considered in the medical treatment of the acute illness or reason for admission. This chapter reviews the special challenges of the acutely ill patient with dementia and presents the concept of the specialized Acute Care for Elders (ACE) unit.

THE PATIENT WITH DEMENTIA

The patient with dementia can present in several different ways to the acute care setting. He or she may be admitted for acute illness, and dementia is a new diagnosis made during that admission. The patient may be admitted with an acute illness while in the middle stages of dementia or admitted with end-stage dementia for end-of-life care. Each stage has unique characteristics that must be acknowledged and addressed by the health care team.

New Diagnosis

Consider the patient, Mrs. Jones, who has been admitted to the hospital for a broken hip after a fall at home. Her neighbor found her on the floor the day after her fall. She is 89, widowed with two children, and lives alone. She has been driving her own car, fixing her own meals, and performing her own personal care. The son lives in another state and calls his mother once a month to check in. The daughter lives in the same town as her mother but has a busy life, with a full-time job and two teenaged children. She checks on her mother at least once a week and helps her clean the house and do her laundry. She has noticed that her mother is increasingly forgetful, and she attributes the symptoms to old age.

The admitting team notices that the patient does not seem to understand her medical situation. The social worker talks with the daughter and uncovers the history of a slowly increasing cognitive decline with impairment in independent skills of daily living (particularly money management). The nurses note that Mrs. Jones interacts well with them but has trouble remembering why she is in the hospital and continually forgets how to use her call bell. They wonder if she is able to give informed consent for her surgery. The medical team consults psychiatry to determine Mrs. Jones' capacity for independent decision-making. She is diagnosed with early-stage dementia by the psychiatrists.

Acute Illness in the Already-Diagnosed Person with Dementia

Now, consider Mrs. Smith. She has been living in an assisted living facility because of her cognitive status. Mrs. Smith was diagnosed with dementia four years ago, and the family has noticed a steady decline since then. Staff at the assisted living facility provides her personal care – bathing, dressing, and grooming. She can walk but has poor balance and requires supervision to prevent falls. Mrs. Smith can feed herself once her food is placed in front of her. She interacts with staff, recognizes her daughters, and enjoys visiting with other residents at her facility. She can no longer remember how to use the telephone, and, in fact, cannot learn new tasks, such as using a walker properly. Her eldest daughter has been appointed the power of attorney for both health care and business decisions. This daughter makes decisions with the input of her siblings.

Mrs. Smith is admitted to the hospital with an acute exacerbation of heart failure. Her daughters, who came with her to the emergency room, leave at 9 P.M. when visiting hours end. They feel that Mrs. Smith has settled in, is as comfortable as possible, and that the nurses are able to meet their mother's needs. They kiss their mother goodnight, and leave. A few minutes later, Mrs. Smith becomes agitated and combative. She screams when staff tries to draw her blood. She continually calls out for her daughters and accuses staff of putting her in jail. At 1 A.M., she falls while getting out of bed and fractures her hip.

The Patient with End-Stage Dementia

Mr. Taylor is admitted to the hospital with aspiration pneumonia. He has been living in a nursing home for the past two years. He receives total care at the nursing home and has been bedridden for about two months. His family relates a history of gradual decline over the past seven years. Mr. Taylor no longer recognizes his family, can no longer feed himself, and is incontinent of bowel and bladder. Most of the time, he sleeps. The nursing home staff reports that, over the past three months, Mr. Taylor has had more frequent episodes of choking and coughing when they feed him, as well as progressive weight loss. Last night, he spiked a fever and could not be roused. He was brought to the hospital by ambulance, and his admitting work-up revealed malnutrition and pneumonia, as well as dehydration. Mr. Taylor's daughters request that "everything possible" be done for their father. The son has power of attorney for health care decisions for Mr. Taylor. He lives several hundred miles away, rarely sees his father, and handles most affairs by telephone. His decisions are frequently in conflict with his sisters, who live in close proximity to their father.

Issues of Care

Each of the preceding cases presents distinct but not unusual challenges to the health care team. Although all three patients have dementia, the issues at each stage of dementia are unique.

Early Interventions

Early diagnosis is essential for ensuring effective planning for the future. Early diagnosis can help reduce future medical costs, allow the family time for adjusting to the diagnosis, and allow time for anticipating future needs. Early diagnosis also promotes ongoing, proactive screening to facilitate early implementation of pharmacological and psychosocial treatments, which may help slow decline and prevent associated disorders such as depression and agitation.

In the first case, the health care team and Mrs. Jones' children have many decisions to make. Is Mrs. Jones able to make her own health care decisions at the present time, based on understanding of the risks and benefits of treatment? In other words, does she have capacity for decision-making? If not, who should make the decisions for her? Should she at least have some input into health care decisions that affect her? Should Mrs. Jones have surgery, based on the risks and benefits presented by the medical team? Who can consent for the surgery and make other health care decisions in the short term? What if the children disagree about treatment for the broken hip?

There are also longer-term issues in this case. What does the future hold for Mrs. Jones? Will she be able to make her own decisions in the future? Can Mrs. Jones return to her previous lifestyle after surgery and rehabilitation? What if she does not have surgery – will this change the discharge plan? Are there safety issues making discharge to home challenging? If she cannot go home, what type of environment will be most appropriate? What kind of care can Mrs. Jones afford? What does the future hold for Mrs. Jones, what decisions about her future can be made now, and what decisions can her children be expected to make in the future? What education is needed for the family and for Mrs. Jones about dementia and the long-term outcomes?

Mrs. Smith has different issues. Her life as a person with dementia has been handled very well. She lives in a setting that is appropriate to her abilities, with supervision and personal assistance as needed. She is safe within that setting but has a limited ability to learn new tasks. Her family is available and supportive. The change in setting from her familiar environment to the hospital caused confusion and fear, leading to the fall and broken hip. And now, the hip fracture itself presents challenges.

Immediate issues include questions such as: Will Mrs. Smith survive surgery? Will she be able to learn, remember, and maintain the safety precautions required after hip surgery? Will hip surgery, a major risk in itself, improve her life? Or would avoiding surgery altogether and providing pain management lead to the best quality of life for Mrs. Smith? How will her heart failure influence her surgical outcome? How can the health care provider assist the patient and her family to make these hard decisions?

And then there is Mr. Taylor, who has been living with dementia for a number of years. The decisions at the end-of-life are different, and in many ways more challenging. What should be done about family disagreements regarding provision of care? If the aspiration pneumonia is related to oral feedings, should alternative routes of feeding (i.e., nasogastric or surgically inserted feeding tubes) be attempted? Can aspiration pneumonia even be prevented with tube feedings? What does the family need to know about end-stage dementia? When should treatment be stopped and natural death encouraged? Is it reasonable and ethical to do "everything possible" for Mr. Taylor?

The health care team is an important part of dementia care in the acute care setting. They must be ready to consider the entire bio-psycho-social characteristics of the patient, recognize the unique aspects of each stage of dementia, and provide expert discharge planning, education, and family support. It has been recognized that these are difficult tasks that many providers are not ready to meet. The ACE model of care fits well with this patient population.

THE ACE UNIT

The Acute Care for Elders (ACE) concept is a model of care that is gaining in popularity in the United States. Just as the Eden Alternative has caused us to change the environment of nursing homes to a more home-like setting, acute care hospitals must examine the environment they provide for the hospitalized elderly patient. The ACE model specifically addresses the needs of the hospitalized older adult. The purpose of an ACE unit is to prevent the complications of hospitalization in a home-like setting with highly trained staff, while addressing the bio-psycho-social needs of the patient and family. It is a model of care that fits well with the person with dementia, no matter the stage of his or her disease. Environment, staff expertise, and the interdisciplinary team are three key aspects of the ACE Unit (Table 10.1).

Environment is one of the most important aspects of ACE. De-institutionalizing the appearance of the inpatient geriatric unit, while meeting the needs of the acute care staff, is a central goal of environmental adaptation. Carpeting, to decrease visual glare and noise, and to soften falls, decreases the institutional look of the hospital. A living room offers an area to eat meals, socialize with others, and engage in therapeutic recreation. Age-appropriate paintings on the walls make the area more home-like. The nurses' station becomes a formal reception area to the unit,

TABLE 10.1 Key Elements of an ACE Unit

Elements	Goal	Examples
Appropriate physical environment	To promote safety and independence	Handrails in halls, noise control, good lighting, carpeting, nonskid flooring, homelike atmosphere
Patient-centered care	To identify and minimize common geriatric problems while enhancing nutrition and other health factors	Evidence-based protocols that address nutrition, sleep, mobility, falls, and other geriatric-specific issues
Medical care	To identify and prevent medical problems common to hospitalized older adults	Attention paid to constipation, delirium, pain, polypharmacy, and other common problems
Discharge planning	To identify patient's future needs and level of care after the hospitalization	Interdisciplinary teamwork

while the nurses perform their work closer to patients' rooms. Windows in the hallways allow patients to be seen in their rooms, which increases socialization and helps to prevent falls. Hospital equipment is hidden from view to decrease the hospital-like atmosphere. Handrails and handicap-accessible bathrooms encourage out-of-bed activity. Large bedrooms with sleeper sofas encourage the family to stay with the patient and help to provide a familiar, friendly, family-like atmosphere (Figure 10.1).

Highly trained staff is also core to the ACE concept. Staff is trained in geriatrics as well as individual specialties. Staff education is ongoing in seminars, grand rounds, and in-service training. Staff orientation and competency assessment tools are structured and geriatric-focused. Administrative support is readily available to promote staff education by sending staff to local, regional, and national conferences on geriatrics. Staff members also teach each other during personal encounters or even in team rounds. Many ACE staff members become geriatric-certified within their specialties.

An ACE interdisciplinary team provides for holistic medical, functional, and nursing care. Usual team members include the geriatrician, nurse, pharmacist, physical therapist, occupational therapist, dietitian, and social worker. Other disciplines are available for consult, such as

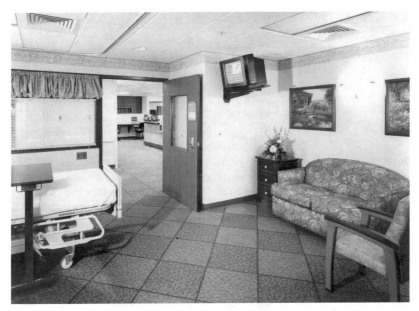

FIGURE 10.1   Bedroom in the ACE unit.

chaplain, speech-language pathologist, and respiratory therapist. The interdisciplinary team (Table 10.2) meets regularly to discuss patient management and discharge planning. Volunteers also staff the unit, assisting with therapeutic recreation and visiting with patients.

Preventing geriatric syndromes is at the heart of interdisciplinary team activity. Geriatric syndromes include such complications of hospitalization as delirium, falls, pressure ulcers, and malnutrition. Protocols such as those recommended by NICHE (Nurses Improving Care for Health System Elders, a John A. Hartford Foundation program described in Chapter 9) are used to standardize care given by the team (Table 10.3). Every effort is made to de-institutionalize the setting and hospital routines. Thus, on ACE, all staff members encourage out-of-bed activity. Group activities in the living room, walking in the hall with staff, and going to the PT gym are all appropriate ACE activities. Confused patients are included in all social activities. Music therapy through activities like listening to CDs, singing, or playing piano becomes part of hospital care. Pet therapy is provided on many ACE Units through fish tanks of colorful fish and therapy dogs. Falls are prevented through strengthening programs, out-of-bed activities, and prevention of delirium. Pressure ulcers are prevented through out-of-bed activities and close surveillance of skin condition. And mealtimes become social events for some patients, increasing the likelihood of adequate intake.

TABLE 10.2 The ACE Interdisciplinary Team

Team member	Primary role(s)
Physician	Manage the medical aspects of the patient's care, assist in discharge planning
Nurse	Assess patient's physical and functional status, deliver basic nursing care, implement physician orders, educate patient and caregiver, fall prevention, assist with discharge planning
Social worker	Assess home situation, screen for abuse and neglect, assist with advance directives, facilitate a safe discharge to the least restrictive and most appropriate environment, assist with accessing community resources
Physical therapist	Assess mobility, prescribe mobility aids such as canes and walkers, prescribe and teach strengthening exercises for the lower limbs, initiate fall prevention activities, educate patient and caregiver, recommend discharge environment
Occupational therapist	Assess ability to perform activities of daily living (bathing, dressing, grooming, feeding self), assess cognition, prescribe and teach exercises to improve self care activities, recommend discharge environment
Pharmacist	Review medications, assist physicians with ordering age-appropriate medications, educate family and caregivers, assist with accessing community resources for medication costs
Dietitian	Assess nutritional status, recommend alternatives to diet to maintain caloric intake, educate patient and caregiver
Speech language pathologist	Assess safety of swallowing of food and fluids; assess communication techniques; recommend interventions based on assessments

THE ACE UNIT AND THE PERSON WITH DEMENTIA

The ACE concept of acute care presents an opportunity to better treat the hospitalized person with dementia. To carry the above case studies a bit further, ACE team strategies are presented for Mrs. Jones, Mrs. Smith, and Mr. Taylor.

TABLE 10.3 Examples of ACE Interdisciplinary protocols

Protocol	Purpose	Primary team members involved in implementation of protocol
Abuse and neglect	Screening, recognition, prevention, intervention for abuse and/or neglect	Nursing, social worker, physician, others as indicated
Advance directives	Educating patient and family about, and facilitating implementation of, advance directives	Nursing, social workers, physician
Behavior management	Prevention of agitated behavior, harm to patient or others	Nursing, physician, PharmD, PT, OT
Bowel and bladder management	Prevention of constipation, management of incontinence, prevention of infection, education of caregivers	Nursing, physician, Pharm-D, OT, social worker
Cognitive assessment	Assessing baseline cognitive status and recognizing variations from baseline	Nursing, physician, OT, PT, SW, PharmD
Delirium	Prevention and/or early recognition of confusion	Physician, nursing, PT, OT, PharmD
Depression	Early recognition and treatment of depressive symptoms	Physician, nursing, PharmD, PT, OT, SW
Discharge planning	Planning and executing a discharge to the least restrictive, safest, and most appropriate environment	Social worker, nursing, PT, OT, physician
Fall prevention	Prevention of falls	Nursing, PT, OT, SW, PharmD, physician
Functional assessment	Assessing baseline functional status	Nursing, PT, OT, physician
Nutrition	Ensuring adequate intake and safe swallowing	Nursing, physician, OT, SLP, dietitian
Pain management	Ensuring adequate recognition of and treatment for pain	Nursing, physician, PharmD, PT, OT
Polypharmacy	Limiting medications to the fewest and safest	Physician, PharmD, Nursing
Pressure ulcer prevention	Prevention of bedsores	Nursing, PT, OT

Mrs. Jones

Mrs. Jones is admitted to the ACE Unit from the emergency room with a broken hip. Within the first 24 hours on the unit, thorough assessments are completed by the geriatric physician, orthopedic surgeon, nurse, and

social worker. The physical and occupational therapists, recognizing
that Mrs. Jones' postoperative picture may look very different from her
current state, speak briefly to her and her daughter about the home situation. They delay further assessment until the first day postop, but do
introduce the idea of a posthospital stay in a skilled nursing facility or
rehabilitation facility, depending on recovery from surgery. The dietitian
reviews Mrs. Jones' laboratory work-up, and speaks with the patient
and daughter about Mrs. Jones' usual nutritional intake.

The geriatric physician orders a medical work-up based on Mrs.
Jones' age, anticipated surgical risks, and current medical status. The
ACE team pays particular attention to cardiac and pulmonary status,
since heart and lung function is very important to a successful surgery.
An EKG, chest X-ray, and stress test are ordered to ensure that these
body systems are functioning well. They also order laboratory work to
rule out anemia, infections, electrolyte imbalances, and nutritional deficits. Laboratory work is also ordered to check Mrs. Jones' blood clot-
ting status, since she has been on anticoagulants for atrial fibrillation.
The geriatric physicians implement orders to prevent common geriatric
syndromes: pain medication, laxatives as needed, a regular diet, preventive medications for deep vein thrombosis, and her usual medications for
hypertension and atrial fibrillation. They stop the anticoagulants that
she was taking for her atrial fibrillation, in anticipation of surgery. The
geriatricians also assess Mrs. Jones cognitive status, and her ability to
make her own health care decisions.

The orthopedic surgeon reviews the X-rays of Mrs. Jones' hip taken
in the emergency room to plan for the surgery. A tentative surgical date
is chosen, and the surgery is scheduled with the operating room. Consents are obtained from Mrs. Jones for surgery, since the geriatricians
have deemed her cognitively intact.

In the first 24 hours, the ACE nurses also assess Mrs. Jones. They
identify that she is at risk for falls, pressure ulcers, delirium, pain, and
constipation, and they implement written plans of care for each of these
issues. The nurses educate the patient and daughter about anticipated
pre- and postoperative routines, such as recovery room, a possibility of
a short ICU stay, and gradually increasing activity postop. They, too,
broach the topic of a posthospital stay in a skilled nursing or rehabilitation facility. The nurses communicate with the social workers and
therapists their concerns about the patient returning to her own home,
because she has a pressure ulcer on her nonoperative hip from laying on
the floor after her fall.

The pharmacist reviews the patient's prehospitalization medication
list, and compares it to the physicians' inpatient orders. She discusses
alternatives to warfarin, Mrs. Jones' anticoagulant, with the physicians.

She also reviews the patient's renal function, and reminds the physicians of medications that have been ordered that may not be appropriate due to her aging kidneys. The pharmacist relates concerns about Mrs. Jones' ability to maintain an effective medication regimen at home, due to her forgetfulness and inability to remember the names of her home medications.

The ACE team meets daily to discuss their patients, and to collaborate in plans for patients' discharges. All team members participate in the rounds, voicing their assessments and worries about patient progress and discharge. Mrs. Jones has surgery, progresses through ACE physical and occupational therapy, and receives recommendations from the therapists that she go to a rehabilitation facility for intensive therapy. The physician reports the diagnosis of early dementia and requests that the team help educate the patient and family about the implications of this diagnosis in regard to function and discharge planning. The social worker discusses the patient's and family's wishes about an appropriate facility and makes formal referrals to these facilities for the patient. The social worker also meets often with the patient and family to discuss the diagnosis of dementia and to recommend considerations to the patient and family for planning Mrs. Jones' future, such as completion of advance directives.

Mrs. Jones is discharged from the ACE unit to a rehabilitation facility. The ACE team has helped her and her family adjust not only to the pre- and postoperative phases of hip surgery; they also have prevented geriatric syndromes during the hospitalization. The ACE team has helped the patient and family adjust to the diagnosis of early dementia, identified useful community resources, and taught them about what to expect as the dementia advances. Advance directives have been completed, and the daughter has been formally identified as the power of attorney for health care. The ACE team feels that this is a safe discharge, that appropriate follow-up care is planned, and that the patient and family have been well educated. The patient and family are highly satisfied with their inclusion in health care planning and decisions, and feel comfortable that they can address the responsibilities before them.

Mrs. Smith

Mrs. Smith had a routine admission to the ACE unit before her fall. She was seen and assessed by the geriatrician, nurse, physical therapist, occupational therapist, dietitian, and pharmacist. Issues pertaining to her congestive heart failure were addressed, such as chest X-ray, EKG, medication review, and relief of her fluid overload. Geriatric syndromes were addressed, with orders for prevention of constipation, DVT, and orders for out-of-bed activity. Plans of care were initiated for nutrition, prevention of delirium, falls, and pressure ulcers.

After her fall, other measures were put into place by the ACE interdisciplinary team. Mrs. Smith was moved to a large room, which facilitated family involvement in her care. Because she exhibited fear of the unknown and of strange staff, her daughters were encouraged to stay with her as much as possible, even through the night. Orthopedics was consulted to evaluate the possibility of hip surgery. A family meeting was held with the team and daughters to discuss realistically the options for care: surgery versus no surgery. The risks of surgery would be age related, with even more risks due to the dementia. Inability to learn the weight-bearing status required after hip surgery could lead to failure of the surgery, or increased bed rest with the accompanying risks of pneumonia, deep vein thrombosis, or pressure ulcers. Risks of nonsurgery include ongoing pain, bed rest until healing occurs, and discharge to a more restrictive facility.

Discussions were also held with the family about plans for end-of-life care. The orthopedic surgeons determined that some weight bearing would be possible after surgery, so the daughters decided that Mrs. Smith would undergo hip repair. The daughters expressed great satisfaction with the care that their mother received, and particularly appreciated the open communication about realistic risks and benefits of treatment. They also appreciated the opportunity and invitation to participate in their mother's care.

Mr. Taylor

The ACE team went into immediate action with Mr. Taylor. The team assessments revealed a patient in end-stage dementia, where the ability to eat was greatly impaired due to the disease process. The team knew that eating and swallowing difficulties were signs of end-stage dementia. They knew that the research literature showed that artificial routes of feeding in people with dementia did not prolong life or change outcomes in persons at this stage of life. Specifically, they knew that research had shown that artificial feeding in the end stages of dementia cannot reverse malnutrition and weight loss, prevent pressure ulcers, prevent aspiration pneumonia, or improve quality of life. In fact, artificial feeding has been found to decrease the quality of life by increasing the probability of physical or chemical restraints aimed at preventing the patient from pulling out the tube. Also, there are always potential complications from tube insertion such as pain and infection, and the ever-present risk of tube malfunction. Thus, risks outweigh the benefits in terms of artificial feeding in the patient with end-stage dementia (Li, 2002).

The social worker spoke with the patient's son, the power of attorney for health care, and learned that he did not want heroic or extensive measures taken to prolong his father's life. He said that his father expressed that he never wanted to be a vegetable, and if he were not able to enjoy life, he would rather die. The son felt he was honoring his father's wishes by validating a Do Not Resuscitate order, and refusing artificial feedings. He did approve comfort feeding (eating food as desired in the normal manner by mouth), with the knowledge that it could hasten death from aspiration pneumonia.

The ACE team gained permission from the son to have a family meeting with the daughters. The meeting was held, and staff educated the daughters about the potential and very realistic outcomes for Mr. Taylor. When the daughters challenged the son's right to make decisions, the social worker related the meaning of the power of attorney for health care documents, as well as Mr. Taylor's wishes for a good death. It was decided, with input from the daughters and decisions from the son, to provide intravenous fluids and antibiotics, to treat acute issues, to provide comfort feedings, and then to send Mr. Taylor to the nursing home with hospice. The family felt comfortable with this decision and expressed appreciation for the ACE team's facilitation of communication between the family members.

A TYPICAL ACE UNIT

ACE units are growing in number. A recent study found sixteen ACE units in the United States (Jayadevappa, Bloom, Raziano, & Lavizzo-Mourey, 2003), although others have reported that there are more than one hundred (Li, 2003). ACE units can be found in both teaching and private hospitals, in both community and urban settings. Clinical outcomes from ACE units, such as complication rates, length of stay, and function have been reported to be better than usual medical care. For instance, Landefeld, Palmer, Kresevic, Fortinsky, and Kowal, (1995) report improvement in ADL function, ability to walk, symptoms of depression, and nursing home placement in patients after ACE unit admissions. Counsell et al. (2000) report improvements in processes of care, including reductions in restraint use and fewer prescriptions of high-risk medications.

Standard care for the hospitalized geriatric population is based on traditional care that has evolved over the past half century and does not take into consideration the needs of the geriatric population. Standard care was developed and provided in a disease-based model of all age groups. Using the standard model of care sets up the geriatric patient for complications, extended lengths of stay, and a higher number of transfers to long-term care facilities, thus contributing to a downward functional spiral that results in bad outcomes for the patient and an economic burden for the hospital.

The ACE unit at the University of Texas Medical Branch (UTMB) in Galveston is a geriatric-friendly environment. Situated in a 700-bed university teaching hospital, the homelike environment, the staff, and the interdisciplinary team have all been in place since 2000. Funding from the Sealy-Smith Foundation provided renovations to make the unit patient and nurse friendly. Nurses, therapists, social workers, and a PharmD (as well as Tilly, the therapy dog) all report to a single Director of Geriatrics. More than 65% of nurses are certified in geriatrics, as are the PharmD and one of the physical therapists. The interdisciplinary team meets daily, Monday through Friday, to discuss each patient on the twenty-bed unit. Family meetings are common, and open communication is stressed.

Interdisciplinary teamwork is continual. Not only does the team see the patients, they also work together through shared governance and continuous process improvement on systems and procedural issues. The interdisciplinary team is examining such issues as falls, care planning, and pressure ulcer prevention together.

The ACE unit is a twenty-bed medical surgical nursing unit. The primary criteria for admission is that the patient be age 65 or older. The only exclusionary criteria that exist are need of critical care, an acute myocardial infarction, and the need of oncological medications best given by a specially trained nursing staff. Therefore, the case mix on the ACE unit, with the exceptions noted above, is essentially the same as would be found for a 65-year-old on any medical surgical unit in any hospital.

Between 30 and 60% of the UTMB ACE unit's patients are admitted with dementia as either a primary or secondary diagnosis. The interdisciplinary team continually works together to address the complex bio-psycho-social needs of these patients. Because the hospital is located on a small barrier island, staff has a unique opportunity to get to know their patients, to monitor them over time, and to help both patient and family adjust to the diagnosis and processes of dementia. The ACE unit environment helps to facilitate the delivery of care to this population.

There are many factors that set the UTMB ACE model of care apart from standard care. For instance, the usage of geriatric-unfriendly medications such as diphenhydramine and meperidine are lower on this unit than for other comparable patients housewide. Therapists work with approximately 70% of all ACE patients compared to 21% of elderly patients on other units. The fact that the nurses are certified in geriatric nursing demonstrates that they are well educated in the management of the older adult, including patients with delirium and dementia. Patient satisfaction is high on the UTMB ACE unit, and staff turnover is negligible. Since the unit opened, RN vacancies have been filled immediately. Outcomes have been so remarkable that the hospital administration has approved adding another thirty-two ACE beds in 2005.

Outcomes for the ACE unit at UTMB have been positive in terms of quality of care and economic measures. The ACE unit has demonstrated a decreased length of stay (LOS), case-mix adjusted, as compared to standard care hospital care (case-mix adjusted LOS is the length of stay weighted by the severity of illness). This decrease in LOS does not increase the patient's readmission rate or result in an increase in transfers to long-term facilities. This is an important indicator of economics for hospitals. The rule of thumb is that as the case-mix number increases, so does the resource utilization and reimbursement. The goal of the hospital, therefore, is to care for patients as efficiently as possible so that the resource utilization does not outstrip the reimbursement. This goal is also in the best interest of the patient. A shorter LOS results in fewer complications of the hospital stay for the patient, generally less debilitation, and a higher quality of life posthospitalization.

Although the ACE model of care has been successful at UTMB, challenges remain. Informal conversation among professionals who work in ACE units across the United States reveals a common ongoing challenge of communicating the philosophy of ACE care with physicians who are not geriatricians, yet who care for patients on ACE units. Often, these physicians were not exposed to interdisciplinary teamwork in their training, so they are not prepared to interact with the ACE team. Also, there is much work to be done on benchmarking ACE unit outcomes across ACE units in the United States and abroad. Luckily, communication networks are being forged among ACE units to work on issues that are similar across settings.

CONCLUSION

The ACE unit concept can more than adequately serve the patient with dementia, no matter the stage. The homelike environment, staff knowledgeable in geriatric care, and the interdisciplinary team can all focus attention on the needs of the patient, rather than being distracted by other issues.

Of course, the population of older adults with dementia is not the only population that can benefit from the ACE model of care. Older adults, particularly those over 85, often present to the acute care hospital environment with complex needs. Social issues concerning living arrangements, end-of-life issues, advance directives, finances, and changes within the structure of the family can add a burden to the typical acute care environment. The medical picture is often complex, with an acute illness superimposed on multiple chronic illnesses, with resultant changes in function and ability to care for self. The psychological picture is clouded with normal reactions to changing social situations and physical health. The ACE unit offers a model of care and staff who are prepared to offer expert and specialized assistance to help the older adult address the inevitable complex issues associated with aging.

REFERENCES

Counsell, S. R., Holder, C. M., Liebenauer, L. L. Palmer, R. M. Fortinsky, R. H., Kresevic, D. M., Quinn L. M., Allen, K. R., Corinsky, K. E., & Landefeld, C.S. (2000). Effects of a multi-component intervention on functional outcomes and process of care in hospitalized older patients: A randomized controlled trial of Acute Care for Elders (ACE) in a community hospital. *Journal of the American Geriatrics Society, 48,* 1572–1581.

Jayadevappa, R., Bloom, B. S., Raziano, D. B., & Lavizzo-Mourey, R. (2003). Dissemination and characteristics of acute care for elders (ACE) units in the United States. *International Journal of Technology Assessment in Health Care. 19*(1), 220–227.

Landefeld, C. S., Palmer, R. M., Kresevic, D. M., Fortinsky, R. H., & Kowal, J. (1995). A randomized trial of care in a hospital medical unit especially designed to improve the functional outcomes of acutely ill older patients. *New England Journal of Medicine, 332,* 1338–1344.

Li, I. (2002). Feeding tubes in patients with severe dementia. *American Family Physician, 65*(8), 1605–1610.

Li, J. (2003). Focus on Quality: from a Report on the Society of Hospital Medicine 6th Annual Meeting. Medscape Conference Coverage. Retrieved January 4, 2005, from http://www.medscape.com/viewarticle/456550

CHAPTER 11

Windows to the Heart

Creating an Acute Care Dementia Unit[1]

Jeffrey N. Nichols

In 1999, Cabrini Medical Center, a 500-bed hospital in New York City, received a grant from the United Hospital Fund to create a family-centered acute care unit for patients with dementia. Because of its location in lower Manhattan, the hospital serves an ethnically diverse population, including many non-English-speaking people of Hispanic and Asian origin. It also has a high proportion of elderly patients, including patients with dementia.

The eight-bed acute care unit was intended to address the widely recognized problem that when people with dementia are hospitalized, the experience is often highly stressful for both the patient and the family or nonkin caregivers. Patients with advanced Alzheimer's disease and other dementias often suffer a precipitous decline in function during and after hospitalization, which places additional burdens on both the patients and their caregivers. Following focus group research with family caregivers of patients with dementia, senior hospital administrators decided that it would not be sufficient to "tweak this, tweak that" in the traditional system of care in order to meet the identified needs. Rather, it

---

[1]This chapter is adapted with permission from an interview conducted by Karen S. Heller with the author, soon after the unit opened in early 2000, and published in *Innovations in End-of-Life Care* (Romer et al., 2002) and in the *Journal of Palliative Medicine* (Nichols & Heller, 2002).

would be necessary to take a comprehensive, carefully orchestrated, and holistic approach to change—encompassing the physical, operational, and cultural environment of the institution.

This chapter describes the challenges faced in starting the acute care dementia unit and provides some preliminary evidence for its value. The chapter includes the author's observations and insights about the unit after five years of operation.

GENESIS OF THE PROJECT

The project, which was called "Windows to the Heart," began in response to a grant program launched by the United Hospital Fund to enable New York City hospitals to look at ways they could support family caregivers. Because Cabrini's elderly patient population includes many patients with dementia, the hospital decided to target family caregivers of these patients. The exact proportion of patients with dementia in the hospital's patient population was not known, but staff believed it was significant. Unfortunately, most hospitals do not do good screening, and hospital data systems are not designed to capture information about dementia, which is usually not the patient's primary diagnosis. About 70% of residents of Cabrini's affiliated nursing home have dementia, however, and the nursing home supplied a portion of admissions to the hospital. In addition, hospital staff believed there were many people with dementia living in the community surrounding the hospital.

Cabrini applied for and received an initial planning grant from the United Hospital Fund in 1998. A project advisory panel was formed with representatives from hospital administration, the hospital's medical and nursing staff, and the New York City Alzheimer's Association Chapter, as well as two family caregivers.[2] The advisory panel decided to conduct some focus groups of family caregivers who had had a relative admitted to Cabrini. Nursing staff identified patients they could remember in the previous few months whose care had involved family caregivers. These family caregivers were invited to share their experiences and suggestions about hospital care for patients with dementia.

---

[2]Chapter 13 in this volume discusses the perspectives of the New York City Alzheimer's Association Chapter on the need for the Cabrini project and the deliberations of the project advisory panel (Levine & Marks, 2005).

HOSPITALIZATION—"NOT GOOD" FOR PATIENTS WITH DEMENTIA

The focus groups were run by professional focus group coordinators. The advisory panel expected the family caregivers to say they needed support groups, more flexible visiting hours, better information about the disease, and better referrals at the time of discharge. While those needs were mentioned, an even more loud and clear message was that the hospital experience itself was *not good* for the person they loved or for them. Focus group participants said they felt ignored when they came to the hospital. They said they knew crucial things about what the patient needed, but no one asked for or seemed interested in this information. They stated emphatically that hospital personnel were insensitive to the emotional stress they were undergoing and that what they would really like is for the hospital to take better care of the patients.

The family caregivers were very straightforward that Cabrini was not *worse* than other hospitals, but that *every* hospital was bad. Many of them had also had their family members at other hospitals. Cabrini is located in a cluster of hospitals in lower Manhattan which is known in the community as "Bedpan Alley," because there are literally thousands of hospital beds within a couple of square miles. Manhattan is terribly overbedded, and it is sometimes a matter of chance where an ambulance will take a patient.

The literature about hospitalization for patients with dementia, primarily with Alzheimer's disease, shows that patients suffer significant functional decline associated with acute hospital care. The assumption of inevitable functional decline was the received wisdom in the field and had largely been taken for granted. Functional decline was seen as something that had to happen because it is part of the disease. For many people with dementia, going into the hospital was a disaster; they wound up worse off than when they came in. Certainly, anyone who has worked in a nursing home will say that patients always come back from the hospital in worse shape than when they left.

Now, in the focus groups, families were saying exactly the same thing. They brought in a person who was moderately functional but had an acute medical problem, usually unrelated to dementia; when the person came out of the hospital, the acute medical problem was improved, but the person's functional status was dramatically worse. Moreover, in the course of the hospitalization, both the family and the patient went through some humiliating experiences.

Given these responses from families and other information gathered in the year-long planning period, the advisory panel recommended that the hospital create a special unit for patients with dementia who were admitted with any of a wide variety of acute medical problems. They recommended that the new unit focus on changing the hospital experience for patients *and* their families.

HOSPITAL RESPONSE TO
RECOMMENDATIONS FOR CHANGE

A combination of factors made Cabrini's senior administrators receptive to the advisory panel's recommendations. The United Hospital Fund's Family Caregiver Initiative was an incentive for the hospital to choose family caregivers' needs as an area on which to focus in the short run. When foundations fund initiatives, they are able to bring attention to an issue. An institution may decide to focus on that issue or not, but the foundation interest directs people and institutions to *think* about the issue.

A second factor that really made a difference was that some of the hospital's senior administrators were caregivers themselves, and some of their loved ones had been in the hospital. Thus, the stories that came out of the focus groups had a certain resonance for those individuals that they might not have had for others. This was really not so surprising; given the statistics on the proportion of middle-aged people who are family caregivers, one would expect that at practically every hospital, there are some senior staff who are also family caregivers. The "Windows to the Heart" project benefited from the fact that senior hospital administrators had had these experiences and consequently supported the project.

Third, Cabrini Medical Center is sponsored by a religious order, the Missionary Sisters of the Sacred Heart of Jesus, known to most people as the Cabrini Sisters. The hospital takes mission issues seriously. Part of its mission is to provide family-centered care and care that is more than just getting people in and out of the hospital. When the hospital's administrators heard family caregivers' stories about difficult hospital experiences for patients with dementia, they agreed that it was important to do something different.

DECISION TO CHANGE THE CULTURE OF CARE

A group of senior administrators from the hospital and its affiliated nursing home met to discuss the focus group findings and advisory panel's recommendations. The more they talked, the clearer it became that the situation could not change in a piecemeal fashion—"tweak this, tweak that, and everything will be all right." In fact, the whole culture of care needed to change, including the way staff interacted with families and the way patients with dementia were cared for in the hospital. This change would affect job descriptions and what was considered important and not important for many hospital staff members. Family caregivers could not be seen as just one more problem in a busy day, which, to a large extent, was the way they were viewed at the time. On a good day, staff might have time to deal with family caregivers' needs, but in a hospital, there are always six billion things to do, and family caregivers' needs often seem like just one more thing on top of everything else. That would have to change.

In 1999, Cabrini applied for and received a second grant from the United Hospital Fund to create an eight-bed acute care unit for patients with dementia. The primary goals for the unit were to change the culture of care for patients with dementia and involve family caregivers. Senior administrators and the project team realized that care would not change with just a patch on top of a bad situation—the patch being a little bit of extra time, especially if the extra time was funded by a grant. Yet the grant provided an important stimulus to begin the change process.

At the start, the hospital's intention was to transform the care of patients who were already using the hospital, rather than to increase referrals of new patients. As the project progressed, the unit staff identified attracting other patients as a potential indicator of success, but the hospital's original goal was to do a better job taking care of its existing patient population.

BARRIERS TO CHANGE AND STRATEGIES FOR OVERCOMING THEM

One barrier the project team thought it would face was a general belief that nothing could ever change, that the way things are is somehow inevitable. The team thought it would eventually be possible to change the culture of care throughout the whole hospital. They knew, however, that changing the culture of care in even one unit would require buy-in from all parts of the hospital, because what was planned would cut across many different boundaries. They thought that if they tried to create a unit that was separate and different, but not accepted by the rest of the hospital, it would ultimately be crushed. For this reason, the team invested a great deal of time in recruiting the interest or at least the understanding of all sorts of people who potentially would be affected by efforts to change the culture of care.

The project team tried very consciously to involve everyone early on, to let them know what was being planned, and to say openly, "These are things that are going to be different; is that all right with you? Is that going to represent a problem? Tell us what the problem is in advance." The team wanted to make sure that everyone whose department was going to be affected had made a commitment in advance, blessed the project, so to speak, and said that it was *all right*, or at least that they were prepared to deal with the reality that it *was not* all right.

The vice presidents for medicine and nursing were recruited because this was going to be a medical unit. Department heads for human resources, food service, pharmacy, housekeeping, social work, discharge planning, chaplaincy, admissions, and security were also recruited. If there were a need to change visiting hours, for example, it would be important to have admissions and security involved.

The project team knew that extra time would be needed from social services. Rather than just scheduling the extra meetings and then hearing from the director of social services, "My staff does not have to come to all these meetings; we have other things to do," the team asked the director of social services, "How much time can you commit for your staff to attend the extra meetings we know are going to be necessary? We are not going to schedule more time than you think they can reasonably provide." With this approach, the director of social services actually committed to a larger number of hours than the project team would have requested. It became an accepted responsibility of social work staff to attend the meetings, and, for a while at least, getting them to attend was not an issue.

Initially, human resources leaders were worried that there might be objections from union personnel about anything that appeared to change job descriptions and reporting. The project team was careful about how these changes were made, and this turned out not to be an issue.

In any large bureaucracy, people who have not been consulted inevitably have concerns that they will want to have addressed later on. If they are involved early in solving the problem, or even framing the problem, they will be much more invested in the success of the project. The time spent initially by the project team to recruit and involve department directors paid off. When these people were asked to identify potential problems, they identified fewer problems, and they were more flexible and more understanding of what the needs were going to be than was originally expected.

DESIGNING THE NEW UNIT

To design the physical layout of the new unit, the project team consulted with Lorraine Hiatt, one of the country's best known experts in dementia design. She spent a day onsite and gave advice on how to make the space responsive to the needs of people with dementia, while working within a limited budget.

The available space was a stretch of rooms that went around a corner at one end of the hospital's sixth floor. The space included four two-bed rooms, a four-bed room in the corner, and a nursing station. To create the new unit, the corner room was converted into a caregiver and patient lounge. The beds and existing wall equipment in that room were replaced with couches and a chair that folds out into a bed. A lot of small tables were placed in the lounge because dementia patients tend to eat better in a social setting. Shelves were added for patient education materials. A wheelchair-accessible bathroom and a family caregiver bathroom were added. Carpet was placed in the lounge and hallways, with prior approval from the hospital's infection control staff. The project team had been warned that some of these changes, especially the carpet, would be difficult to get approved, but this also turned out not to be an issue.

The four two-bed rooms stayed almost exactly as they had been before. They were repainted to more neutral colors, and the lighting was upgraded because shadows and odd lighting situations tend to induce paranoia and fear in patients with dementia.

One basic principle of Alzheimer's design is to make things *look* as much as possible like what they are supposed to be. Doors should look like doors, and outlining the door in color helps people recognize that the door is, in fact, a door. Things that one does not want people to notice should be the same color as the background so they do not stick out. These design principles were followed as closely as possible. The stairwell that goes down to the street is painted the same color as its background wall, with no outlining. All other areas that people are expected to frequent are carefully outlined. Some patients will tend to wander. The general color and layout encourages them to wander in the direction of the caregiver and patient lounge, which is where people are intended to congregate.

TV sets were removed from patient rooms. This might seem almost like a violation of the patient bill of rights, but the project team was aware that loud, confusing, repetitive sounds and hostile images are very difficult for patients with dementia. There is a TV in the lounge, where staff can control what is seen, so patients are not just sitting around with the TV blaring. As a result, the unit is extraordinarily quiet. Music is played. It is not boring, but it is very quiet.

There is limited traffic through the unit because it is in a far corner of the hospital. The only reason to come to the unit is because one wants to be on the unit. No one is wandering through with squeaky carts.

No one is yelling, "Get seventeen out of bed, have to go down to CAT scan," with a patient not knowing whether he or she is number seventeen. There is no distracting overhead paging. The only sounds patients hear are sounds that are *intended*. In addition, efforts are made to bring patients into the lounge, where they can interact with other patients and families in a somewhat more spacious setting than their two-bed room.

STAFFING THE UNIT

When the project began, the objective was to have as little difference as possible in staffing between the new unit and other units in the hospital. Part of the reason for this was purely practical. There is no point in setting up a unit that requires special funding, and then have it disappear after the grant money is gone.

From a nursing point of view, the dementia unit has the same staffing as any other unit in the hospital. In fact, one of the reasons for choosing to create an eight-bed unit was that eight beds per nurse is the standard assignment for registered nurses on the day shift. From the beginning, the dementia unit was staffed primarily with in-house nurses transferred from other units.

Most Cabrini patients have their own private physician, and any physician in the hospital's medicine department can admit a patient to the dementia unit. Since the unit has only eight beds, it does not have its own house staff, i.e., interns and residents. Rather, house staff who provide care on other units in the hospital also provide care for patients on the dementia unit.

Initially, the one difference in staffing between the dementia unit and other units was a pastoral care worker who was assigned almost exclusively to the unit. She was Latin American and bilingual, and she had a lot of interaction with the Spanish-speaking patients and Catholic patients and families from all ethnic groups. The pastoral care worker was the only member of the unit care team whose salary was supported by the project grant.

TRAINING, PLANNING, AND
CARE TEAM DEVELOPMENT

The grant to create the new unit included funding for an extended training period, although "training" is probably the wrong word for the detailed planning and care team development activities that occurred in this period. Achieving the project goals would require creative thought and specific ideas about the needs of patients with dementia and their families. All members of the unit's future care team, from the director of geriatrics to housekeeping staff, were asked to envision how their jobs would be different if they were, in fact, responding to the needs of these patients and families.

Members of the care team considered many tasks involved in daily care. One of the tasks of an environmental aide, for example, is to deliver the meal trays. The care team asked, What was going to be different about delivering meal trays in the new unit versus other units in the hospital? Patients with dementia generally require a long time to eat. Most of them need assistance, and some must be completely hand fed. The team arranged for the new unit to get its meal trays first, and to have them picked up last. This arrangement provided an extra half hour between tray delivery and pickup, which means extra time to feed patients.

During the extended training and planning period, very little time was spent training members of the care team about the causes, physiology, and medical treatment of Alzheimer's disease and other dementias. Over the course of almost a year of weekly meetings, only two hours were spent on these topics. Most hospital staff members do not need to know much about the etiology, pathophysiology, and pharmaceutical treatment of Alzheimer's and other dementias. What they *do* need is the ability to look at a patient with dementia and respond to the patient as an individual; listen to a family caregiver and understand the importance of what the caregiver is saying; regard the patient and caregiver as a unit; and respond to the patient's behavior as meaningful communication that needs to be understood. The extended training period and planning period allowed for the development of a care team with these abilities.

INVOLVING AND SUPPORTING FAMILY CAREGIVERS

Usual care practices on the dementia unit involve and support family caregivers in many ways, including extensive initial and ongoing exchange of information. One reason it is often difficult to provide good care for hospital patients with dementia is that the patients cannot communicate clearly about their needs. If the patient starts rubbing his stomach or pounding the table, the behavior may mean "I need to go to the bathroom," or "I'm bored, I want something to do," or "I'm in pain," or "I'm only comfortable if I have a certain thing around." Before the person was hospitalized, a family member was probably feeding, dressing, bathing, and generally taking care of the person everyday, and in most cases, responding to his or her needs remarkably well. That family caregiver is the best source of information about how the patient usually acts and how to interpret his or her nonverbal behavior. Yet in most hospitals, the family caregiver's knowledge and experience are largely ignored. The one person who has the information hospital staff need to provide the best quality care may be asked for a list of the patient's medications and then essentially dismissed.

Nurses on Cabrini's dementia unit use a very different approach. The first questions they ask when a new patient is admitted to the unit are "Who is the caregiver?" "Who knows what this person could do before, so we have some idea what functions we are supposed to be preserving?" "What is reasonable to expect this patient to be able to do?" "If we have a problem, whom should we call to get more information?" With these questions, they elicit not only problems but also approaches and solutions that have worked at home and suggestions about what should be done if a problem occurs in the hospital.

Unit staff obtain information from family caregivers in various ways. They tend to ask open-ended questions. Family caregivers do not come in neat packages, however, and more structured questions may be needed for some caregivers. Sometimes, the primary family caregiver is present at the time of admission, and it is possible to obtain most of the needed information then. In other cases, the patient may have two or three different caregivers, or there is a family member who supervises and a paid caregiver who is with the patient most of the time at home. In these situations, staff must figure out who the various caregivers are and create opportunities to talk with them.

Asking family caregivers questions about their loved one not only results in valuable information for staff; it also reassures the caregiver that unit staff are interested in learning everything they can about the patient and that they respect the caregiver's knowledge and experience. Through their questions and responses, staff members can further reassure family caregivers that they, the staff, understand dementia and its effects. If a family caregiver says that the patient has a history of wandering, for example, staff respond in a way that conveys their familiarity with and acceptance of this and other behaviors that are common in people with dementia.

An informal log is kept on all patients who are admitted to the dementia unit. The log is shared by the care team but does not become part of the patient's formal hospital record. It is retained on the unit so that if a patient is readmitted, staff do not have to ask the same questions again.

Information exchange is a two-way process, and staff on the dementia unit also try to give family members any information they want or need. In the focus groups, family caregivers had said that one really difficult thing about the hospital was that they could never figure out who was taking care of their loved one. On most hospital units, assignment sheets are not posted; nobody knows other people's names; and nametags are hard to read. Family members often spend long periods of time wandering through the unit, trying to find somebody who knows whether their mother did or did not have breakfast this morning. Did Mom go for a particular test? If Mom went for the test, was it completed, or was it canceled because she was too upset?

Staff on the dementia unit try to make it easy for families to know who is involved in their loved one's care. As noted earlier, the unit is located at one end of a large section of the hospital and is physically separated from the rest of the hospital by its layout and design. If a family member walks onto the unit and sees a member of the staff, that staff member is very likely to be involved in the care of his or her loved one. The only dietician who comes onto the unit is the dietician for the unit. The only social worker who comes on the unit is the social worker for the unit. A unit slogan selected early on by the care team was, "You can ask anybody because we're all involved in the care."

The worst that can happen is that a family member asks somebody who does not know the answer, but that person does know who will have the answer. If the staff member who is delivering the lunch tray does not know what the patient had for breakfast, he or she at least knows who does know, so the family member can be directed appropriately. Responsiveness to family members' requests for information has been a very positive aspect of care on the unit. It has led to more respectful and constructive interactions between staff and families than are common in many acute care settings.

In addition to facilitating staff and family exchanges of information, procedures on the dementia unit create a welcoming atmosphere for families. The unit has unlimited visiting hours; families can come at any time. If they want to spend the night, or feel they should spend the night because the patient needs them, they do not have to get special permission. They can use the foldout bed in the caregiver lounge. There are also cots if caregivers want to stay in a patient's room, but staff discourage this practice unless it is absolutely necessary because there are usually two patients in the room, and the caregiver's presence may disturb the other patient.

When the new unit was being planned, many family members said that they were going to want to spend the night. The project team did not know how much capacity would be needed and actually prepared for three or four caregivers to stay on the same night. It turned out that most family members who said they wanted to spend the night did so because they did not trust the hospital to take care of their loved one.

Once family members recognize that unit staff are well-intentioned and know what they are doing, very few family members decide to stay overnight.

Interestingly, a remarkable number of relationships have developed among families of patients on the unit. Professional care providers tend to think it is all about them, assuming that if family members come to the hospital, they must want to see the professionals. In fact, one of the benefits of the dementia unit for family members is the opportunity to share experiences with other families. Staff also try to provide formal opportunities for families to interact and learn from each other, but the *informal* interactions are at least as valuable for some families. When patients need assistance or reminders with eating, for example, some families will make arrangements with each other—"If you're here this morning to help with my dad, I'll be here this evening to help with your mother."

INDICATORS OF VALUE

As of December 2004, the dementia unit had been functioning for almost five years. That in itself is an indicator of value. When the unit opened in early 2000, staff wondered whether it would be continued after the grant ended. As discussed in the following section, there has been a lot of turnover in hospital leadership since the unit opened. Yet support for the unit has been maintained.

The dementia unit is usually almost full, with seven of its eight beds occupied most of the time. That is another indicator of value, especially in Manhattan's overbedded hospital environment. Average length of stay is ten to eleven days, which is probably shorter than the average for comparable patients in other Cabrini units and other hospitals in the city, although certainly longer than average for older patients in general and patients of any age in other parts of the country.

Patients on the dementia unit receive high quality care that addresses both the acute medical problems that brought them to the hospital and their coexisting dementia. Many of the care practices that are used on the dementia unit are new to the hospital but well known in certain long-term care facilities, for example, nursing homes, assisted living facilities, and adult day centers that have focused for years on providing good dementia care. Almost all the problem-solving and behavioral approaches used on Cabrini's dementia unit are used routinely in these long-term care facilities but generally not in hospitals. Hospitals are often perceived (and perceive themselves) as the top of the care system, and most hospitals have not been willing to listen to what is known in long-term care or to incorporate that knowledge into the hospital's culture and system of care. Much of what appears new and different about Cabrini's dementia unit reflects the successful transfer of good dementia care practices from long-term care to an acute care setting.

No formal research has been conducted on patient outcomes on the dementia unit, but careful observation suggests that patients cared for on the unit do better than patients with dementia on other units in the hospital. Patients on the dementia unit *seem* to experience less loss of functional abilities than similar patients on other units. They *seem* to lose less weight. If they were continent on admission, they *seem* more likely to be continent on discharge, and they *seem* to be physically restrained less often than similar patients on other units. If these observations are correct, the unit is accomplishing what it was intended to accomplish for patients. Again however, no research has been conducted to confirm the observations. Such research is needed but difficult to conduct, in part because of the difficulty of identifying an appropriate control group of patients with dementia from other units in the hospital.

Like patients with dementia, family members seem to do better when their loved one is cared for on the dementia unit versus other units in the hospital. No formal satisfaction survey or other caregiver research has been conducted, but comments from families have been extremely favorable.

Two issues that are often difficult for hospital staff, patients with dementia, and families—pain management and end-of-life care—have generally not been problems on the dementia unit. With respect to pain management, the most common obstacle is lack of recognition that a person with dementia is in pain because the person cannot communicate verbally about the pain. Staff members on the dementia unit are educated to recognize that behavioral symptoms, such as agitation, restlessness, and sleeplessness, are often manifestations of pain in patients with dementia. Very few patients on the unit have had the kind of pain that necessitates the involvement of an anesthesiologist or specialized pain team. Instead, what these patients have generally needed is routine pain management, which can be provided relatively easily on the unit once the pain is recognized.

With respect to end-of-life care, the dementia unit has benefited from Cabrini's well-known hospice, which has an inpatient unit one floor above the dementia unit. Most patients who have died on the dementia unit have died unexpectedly. When the unit care team recognizes that a patient is terminally ill, the family is usually encouraged to enroll the patient in the hospice program. Terminally ill patients who need inpatient care are transferred upstairs to the hospice unit, not so much because the patient care is better but because hospice includes better bereavement services for families.

Staff turnover seems to be lower on the dementia unit than on most other units in the hospital, and this lower turnover is probably another indicator of value. Two of the original nurses, one aide, and one housekeeper from the unit's first care team were still working on the unit after almost five years, and another of the original nurses just resigned a year ago.

In the early planning stage, the project staff hoped that improvements in care practices and the culture of care on the dementia unit would eventually spread through the hospital and result in more appropriate care for patients with dementia on other units as well. Although nurses are generally assigned to the dementia unit on a long-term basis, other hospital staff rotate among different units or routinely provide care for patients on several units. The project team hoped that these other staff members would observe and participate in care practices on the dementia unit and then carry these practices to other units. The extent to which this carryover has actually occurred is unclear, but many staff members are at least aware of the different approach to care on the dementia unit. The hospital's interns and residents recognize, for example, that they are expected to do different things for patients on the dementia unit than in other places in the hospital. They know that when patients in beds six through twenty-one become agitated, they can just order physical restraints. In contrast, if patients in beds twenty-two through thirty (the dementia unit) become agitated, they are supposed to see the patient and find out why he or she is upset. Because of rotating coverage, not every intern and resident is familiar with the unit and its approach to patient care, but many are.

A final indicator of value is the positive responses of people from outside the hospital who have visited the dementia unit over the past five years. These visitors include experts in dementia care, dementia design, and dementia clothing from around the country; staff of the national Alzheimer's Association and local Alzheimer's Association chapters; and administrators and staff from other hospitals and nursing homes. While it is difficult to characterize the culture of care in a hospital unit, many people from the outside who have toured the unit have commented, "Yes, the culture of this unit *feels* like, *smells* like, *looks* like, therefore must *be* the culture of care that is right for patients with dementia and their families."

ONGOING CHALLENGES

After almost five years of operation, the dementia unit faces several ongoing challenges. One of these challenges results from frequent turnover in the hospital's senior leadership. Since 2000, Cabrini has had three

CEOs, three vice presidents for medical affairs, and four vice presidents for nursing. Although this amount of turnover is not unusual in New York City hospitals, it means that continuing efforts are needed to maintain support for the unit.

New administrators are not aware of the dementia unit. They were not involved in the early discussions about problems in hospital care for patients with dementia and their families. They do not necessarily understand the goals of the unit or the changes in care that are needed to achieve those goals. Nor are they aware of or committed to the accommodations that have been made by various departments in the hospital to support the unit's care practices.

Some new administrators are more sympathetic than others to the goals and needs of the dementia unit. Some have different priorities for the hospital and, as a result, when the hospital has been in financial difficulty, the unit has occasionally ended up on the "cut list." To avoid this eventuality, the unit director and care team invested considerable time in the same kinds of efforts that paid off early in the project to create interest and support for the unit among senior administrators. Similar efforts will undoubtedly be needed in the future.

Regular turnover among interns, residents, and private attending physicians also requires ongoing efforts to build awareness of the approach to care on the unit and adherence to its care practices. The unit director and care team conduct grand rounds and in-service training programs for this purpose. These activities are used to emphasize key messages about the goals and culture of care on the unit, e.g., the need to maintain patients' functional abilities and involve and support family caregivers. Most new interns, residents, and private physicians are open to these messages, but not all are equally responsive. Since the unit care team has little real control over what physicians choose to do or not do for patients on the unit, gaining the understanding and buy-in of new physicians will be an ongoing challenge for the team.

Justifying the unit from a cost perspective is another challenge. From the beginning, it was clear that the unit had to be financially self-sustaining from the hospital's point of view. In addition, supporters of the unit hoped to be able to show that units like this could happen without a lot of extra funding, so that other hospitals would think, We can do that. The $175,000 grant from the United Hospital Fund covered most of the expenses for planning and start-up. The grant paid for four consultants, including the design consultant and a facilitator for the team meetings. As noted earlier, the grant paid the salary of the pastoral care worker. It also paid overtime costs to bring in staff from all three shifts so that everyone who would be providing care on the unit could be together in the same room for important planning meetings. The hospital paid for the physical changes to the unit and other start-up expenses totaling about $90,000.

The relative cost to the hospital of ongoing care for patients on the dementia unit versus other hospital units is not known. Calculating relative cost is difficult for the same reason it is difficult to develop accurate information about differences in patient outcomes on the dementia unit versus other units in the hospital, that is, the difficulty of identifying comparable patients from different units. Ultimately, information about the relative cost and outcomes of care for patients with dementia on different units is needed to determine the value of the unit.

A final challenge for the dementia unit and the hospital is to ensure that patients with dementia who are appropriate for the unit are, in fact, admitted to the unit on a timely basis. Many admissions to the unit have occurred because a family member says, "I want that unit I read about in the paper," or "I want the unit my friend's father was on." These admissions reflect positive print coverage and word-of-mouth recommendations for the unit. The problem is that the hospital lacks effective mechanisms for identifying other patients with dementia who should be admitted to the unit.

Most hospital patients with dementia are admitted for an acute medical problem that is not directly related to their dementia; the dementia may not be noted in their medical record, and the admitting physician and admissions staff may not even think of the dementia unit. About a third of the patients admitted to the dementia unit are transfers from another unit in the hospital. Often, a patient with dementia is admitted to the other unit; there is a first, terrible day, during which the patient becomes agitated, begins pulling out his or her IV, and is eventually put in physical restraints. At that point, the family may say, "My Dad was on the dementia unit before. The staff there seemed to know how to deal with his behavior." Alternatively, staff on the other unit may recognize that the patient is appropriate for the dementia unit. Someone says, "This never happens with the patients who are down on the special unit for dementia patients. Why don't we transfer this patient down there?" The patient is transferred, and usually becomes less agitated and easier to care for over the next few days. It would be better, however, if the patient were admitted directly to the dementia unit and did not have to go through that disastrous first day. This would be better not only for the patient but also for the family and for hospital staff members on both units who would not have to cope with so many agitated patients and anxious, often angry, families.

Getting patients with dementia admitted to the dementia unit from the hospital's emergency room has been particularly difficult. Originally, it was hoped that the emergency room would be fully involved in the "Windows to the Heart" project. Family caregivers who had participated in the focus groups at the start of the project said that emergency room care for patients with dementia was not good at Cabrini or any other hospital. Thus, the project team expected to work closely with emergency room staff to improve care for patients with dementia in the emergency room and develop ways of identifying patients who would benefit from admission to the dementia unit. Unfortunately, all the emergency room staff members who had expressed interest in participating in the project left the hospital. During much of the planning period, the emergency room was without a director and very short-staffed administratively. Thus, the emergency room was not part of the planning process.

Since the dementia unit opened, Cabrini has had three emergency room directors. For a time, a social worker was jointly assigned to the unit and the emergency room. He was able to identify patients in the emergency room who would be appropriate for the unit and facilitate their admission to the unit. Even so, he was only in the hospital for one shift, five days a week, and eventually he was reassigned to work full time in the emergency room.

In 2002, the New York City Alzheimer's Association Chapter received a grant to create a training program on dementia for medical personnel in emergency rooms. The Chapter worked with the director of Cabrini's dementia unit to create the training program, and it has been delivered to staff in Cabrini's emergency room and emergency rooms in other hospitals in the city.[3] The training program was well received at Cabrini. As a result of turnover and other factors, however, the problem of identifying emergency room patients who should be on the dementia unit has not yet been resolved.

In addition to problems in identifying patients with dementia who are appropriate for the dementia unit, there is also a problem in determining which people with dementia are not appropriate and, therefore, should not be admitted to the unit. For example, some nursing home residents in the late stages of dementia may be too functionally impaired to benefit from the unit. The challenge for the unit and the hospital is to develop formal policies and procedures to ensure that patients with dementia who are likely to benefit from the unit are admitted.

---

[3]For more information about the training program, see Chapter 13 in this volume (Levine & Marks, 2005).

As of late 2004, a new staff member has been hired whose responsibilities include increasing awareness of the dementia unit both inside and outside the hospital. Her involvement will be helpful in addressing many of the ongoing challenges facing the unit.

CONCLUSION AND RECOMMENDATIONS

The "Windows to the Heart" project was successful in creating what is probably still the only acute care unit for hospital patients with dementia in the United States. The unit has been maintained for almost five years. Although no formal research has been conducted on patient outcomes, experience with the dementia unit certainly shows that functional decline is not inevitable for hospital patients with dementia. Experience with the unit also shows that hospitalization of people with dementia does not have to be as difficult and stressful for their families as was reported by family caregivers in the focus groups. In fact, some family members of patients on the dementia unit probably do not even realize how difficult such hospitalizations can be and often are.

Creating a separate dementia unit is obviously not the only possible approach for improving hospital care for patients with dementia. A single unit cannot possibly provide care for all the patients with dementia in a hospital. Another approach would be to try to change care practices on all units that have patients with dementia. This approach could reduce the problem of getting patients with dementia who could benefit from these care practices admitted to the dementia unit. On the other hand, it is undoubtedly easier to create the kinds of changes that were instituted through the "Window to the Heart" project in a separate unit. This is probably especially true for the environmental design changes and development of the care team, both of which contribute to the culture of care that outside visitors have said *must be right* for patients with dementia and their families.

More important, however, than the decision about whether to create a special unit or try to change care practices on several units at a time is the process through which hospital administrators and staff focus on the needs of patients with dementia and their families and consider how those needs can be met in the context and culture of their acute care setting. The dementia unit's care team continues to struggle against the notion that there are prefabricated solutions for patient problems—something a physician can just "look up" before prescribing or writing orders for care. Instead the team continues to try to persuade new physicians and other hospital staff that it is important to actually see the patient and perhaps even more important to talk to the family caregiver, listen to what the caregiver has to say about the patient, and figure out together how to solve the problem. Rather than coming up with a model of care, the approach at Cabrini has been a problem-solving approach, and that is the approach this author recommends for other hospitals that want to improve care for their patients with dementia.

REFERENCES

Levine, J. A., & Marks, J. (2005). Alzheimer's Association New York City Chapter: Strategies for improving hospital care. In N. M. Silverstein and K. Maslow (Eds.), *Improving Hospital Care for People with Dementia* New York: Springer.

Mace, N. L., & Rabins, P.V. (1999). *The 36 hour day* (3rd ed.). Baltimore, MD: Johns Hopkins Press.

Nichols, J. N. (2002). Windows to the Heart: Creating an acute care dementia unit. In A. L. Romer, K. S. Heller, D. E. Weissman, and M. Z. Solomon (Eds.), *Innovations in end-of-life care* (Vol. 3, pp. 107–124). Larchmont, NY: Mary Ann Liebert Publishers.

Nichols, J. N., & Heller, K. S. (2002). Windows to the Heart: Creating an acute care dementia unit. *Journal of Palliative Medicine* 5(1), 181–192.

Romer, A. L., Heller, K. S, Weisman, D. E., & Solomon, M. Z. (Eds). (2002) *Innovations in end-of-life care* (Vol. 3) Larchmont, NY: Mary Ann Liebert Publishers.

Sager, M. A., & Rudberg, M. A. (1998). Functional decline associated with hospitalization for acute illness. *Clinics in Geriatric Medicine, 14*(4), 669–679.

PART IV

STRATEGIES FOR MAKING A DIFFERENCE

Try This: Best Practices in Nursing Care for Hospitalized Older Adults with Dementia

Cora Zembrzuski, Meredith Wallace, and Marie Boltz

The sheer, ever-increasing number of persons with dementia, combined with the complex medical and social factors impacting care, requires that hospital patients with dementia receive specialized nursing assessment and interventions. To that end, the John A. Hartford Institute for Geriatric Nursing at New York University (Hartford Institute) and the Alzheimer's Association are working together to develop a series of brief documents for nurses, called *Try This: Best Practices in Nursing Care for Hospitalized Older Adults with Dementia*. This *Try This* series is an outgrowth of *Try This: Best Practices in Nursing Care to Older Adults*, also developed by the Hartford Institute, to address nursing issues for the aging population in general.

The goal of both *Try This* series is to provide easily accessible, understood, and implemented knowledge of best practices in the care of older adults and to encourage the use of these best practices by all direct care nurses. Each *Try This* issue contains assessment tools, and some issues also provide evidence-based interventions.

This chapter presents an overview of the rationale for the development of *Try This: Best Practices in Nursing Care for Hospitalized Older Adults with Dementia* and describes the six completed issues and three issues that were in the planning phase as of summer 2004. In addition, pertinent issues from the original *Try This* series are presented because of their relevance to the care of older adults who have cognitive impairments.

RATIONALE FOR *TRY THIS*

Demographic Trends

By the year 2050 in the United States, there will be more adults age 65 and older than children age 0 to 14 years. This unprecedented demographic shift has resulted from many advances in science, including new diagnostic techniques, medications, surgical procedures, immunizations, and health promotion knowledge. Many older adults live healthy, productive lives. However, dementia affects over 15% of those 65 years of age or older, 5% of whom have severe dementia (Horgas, Wahl, & Baltes, 1996). Senile dementia of the Alzheimer's type (AD) is the most common form of dementia and accounts for an estimated 60 to 70% of all dementia cases (Hendrie, 1998). The majority (93%) of patients with AD has at least one comorbid condition, and many (approximately 60%) deal with three or more comorbidities (Volicer & Hurley, 1997). Several diseases and conditions are more common in AD as a consequence of the dementing processes, including respiratory and urinary infections, hip fractures, malnutrition, new onset seizures, and pressure ulcers (Leon, Cheng, & Neumann, 1998).

Issues Related to Nursing Care

Because the majority of acute-care nurses caring for patients with dementia has not had specialized education in gerontologic nursing (Armstrong-Esther, Browne, & McAfee, 1999), they are not prepared to recognize and manage the difficulties people with dementia experience when they are hospitalized. Patients with dementia often have difficulty understanding what is being said as well as expressing themselves in a manner that is understood by others (Norberg, 2001). Attendant anxiety that accompanies short-term memory loss is exacerbated by a disruption in routine and the unfamiliar environment of the hospital and results in "behavior problems." Hospital routines that emphasize efficiency challenge the nurse's ability to assess thoroughly the patient with cognitive loss. Workload and related time constraints also compete with efforts to provide focused assessment and individualized interventions (Eriksson & Britt-Inger-Saveman, 2002). Thus, hospital nurses confronted with the demands of caring for clinically complex, vulnerable populations are further challenged by operational and knowledge deficits.

TRY THIS—AN OVERVIEW

Each issue of *Try This* consists of a one-page description of a problem that affects hospital patients with dementia or older people in general and an instrument or technique to assess the problem and facilitate appropriate management. The back page of each issue presents the instrument or technique for use by nurses caring for these people. *Try This* documents are intended to be brief and easily used by anyone who merely reads the two pages. Thus, they may be used as "20-minute doses" of education for direct care nurses. Early indications suggest that nurses regard these documents as an efficient way to obtain valuable and necessary information. The Hartford Institute has gained permission from the authors of the *Try This* documents so that they may be reproduced from the web or printed for clinical use.

An advisory board of nationally recognized experts in the field of dementia care, appointed by the Hartford Institute and the Alzheimer's Association, guides the development of the new *Try This* series, *Best Practices in Nursing Care for Hospitalized Older Adults with Dementia*. At least two outside experts review and provide feedback on each issue. The advisory board also determines topics and makes final decisions on all manuscripts.

ASSESSMENT OF COGNITION

Assessment of cognition is pivotal in the care of older adults to identify changes, to indicate when treatment is most effective, and to prevent further cognitive and physical decline as a result of delirium and dementia. Many older adults experience minor loss of memory as they age. Normal changes of aging result in diminished blood flow to the brain and loss of neurons that may cause these minor changes. Sudden, new-onset (hours or days) changes in cognitive status may signal the development of disease processes in the older adult, including urinary tract infections or adverse medication reactions. This sudden onset change in mental status is known as delirium. In addition, depression may affect cognition, and the clinical features of depression are often mistaken for dementia. As shown in the following table, onset, duration, attention, and consciousness are distinguishing factors among dementia, delirium, and depression.

The original *Try This* series, *Try This: Best Practices in Nursing Care to Older Adults* includes three issues on instruments to assess cognition: The Mini Mental State Examination, the Confusion Assessment Method, and The Geriatric Depression Scale. These three instruments can be useful for hospital patients with dementia, but the first step for these patients is recognition by hospital staff that the person may have dementia. Thus, the new *Try This* series includes an issue on recognition of dementia.

Try This: Recognition of Dementia in Hospitalized Older Adults

The *Try This* issue discusses problems and approaches in recognition of dementia. It notes that many hospital patients with dementia have never been formally diagnosed. Moreover, even if their dementia has been diagnosed, that diagnosis may not be noted in their hospital record. Hospital patients with dementia are at much higher risk than other hospital patients for delirium, falls, dehydration, inadequate nutrition, untreated pain, and medication-related problems. They are more likely to wander, to exhibit agitated and aggressive behaviors, to be physically restrained, and to experience functional decline that does not resolve following discharge. The *Try This* issue (Mezey & Maslow, 2004) suggests four approaches hospitals can use to increase recognition of dementia in their older patients, in order to lessen or avoid these problems (see Figure 12.1).

TABLE 12.1   Distinguishing Features: Dementia, Delirium, and Depression

	Delirium	Dementia	Depression
Onset	Abrupt	Slow, insidious	Recent, may be associated with loss
Duration	Hours to days	Months to years	Stable, may be worse in the morning
Attention	Impaired	Normal, except severe cases	Usually normal
Consciousness	Reduced, fluctuating	Clear	Clear

Try This: The Mini Mental State Examination (MMSE)

As noted in this issue from the original *Try This* series, there are many brief mental status tests that can be used to assess cognitive abilities in clinical and research settings. The best known testsis the *Mini Mental State Examination* (MMSE) (Folstein, Folstein, & McHugh, 1975) which consists of eleven questions, assesses five aspects of cognition: orientation, registration, attention and calculation, recall, and language, and takes only a few minutes to administer. A score on the MMSE, or any other brief mental status test, can be a useful indicator of a person's current cognitive status, but a single test score cannot show whether the decline in cognitive level that is symptomatic of dementia. Thus, the primary value and intended use of the MMSE in hospital and other clinical settings is in measuring change in cognitive status over time.

Try This: Confusion Assessment Method (CAM)

Delirium refers to a transient state of global cognitive impairment. Between 15% and 60% of older adults experience delirium during acute-care hospitalizations, yet the condition is often not recognized and is misdiagnosed as dementia in up to 70% of cases (Waszynski, 2001). Delirium results in increased length of hospitalization, increased risk of nursing home admission, decreased ability to perform activities of daily living (ADLs), and increased use of chemical and physical restraints (Fick, Agostini, & Inouye, 2002; Inouye, 1998).

To enhance the ability to diagnose delirium promptly and effectively and to differentiate it from dementia, this *Try This* issue (Waszynski, 2001) recommends the use of the Confusion Assessment Method (CAM) (Inouye, Van Dyck, Alessi, Balkin, Siegal, & Horwitz, 1990). The CAM includes a standardized assessment for the presence of cognitive impairment, e.g., reduced ability to maintain attention to external stimuli and and disorganized thinking, with attention to specific features that have the greatest ability to distinguish delirium from dementia, e.g., reduced level of consciousness; perceptual disturbances; disturbance of the sleep-wake cycle; and increased or decreased psychomotor behavior.

Try This: The Geriatric Depression Scale (GDS)

Depression is a major disorder among older adults in general. About 12% of people with dementia have major depression, and almost half

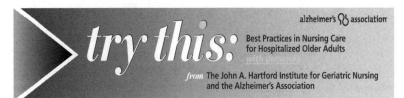

Volume 1, Number 5, Summer 2004   Series Editor: Marie Boltz, APRN, MSN, GNP

Recognition of Dementia in Hospitalized Older Adults

By: Mathy Mezey, EdD, RN, FAAN, and Katie Maslow, MSW

WHY: As many as one third of older hospital patients have dementia. Their dementia may never have been formally diagnosed, and even if it has been diagnosed, the diagnosis may not be noted in their hospital record. Because of stress caused by acute illness and being in an unfamiliar setting, some older patients show symptoms of dementia for the first time in the hospital. Older hospital patients with dementia are at much higher risk than other older hospital patients for delirium, falls, dehydration, inadequate nutrition, untreated pain, and medication-related problems. They are more likely to wander, to exhibit agitated and aggressive behaviors, to be physically restrained, and to experience functional decline that does not resolve following discharge. This *Try This* document suggests ways hospitals can increase recognition of dementia in their older patients, to lessen or avoid any of these problems.

TARGET POPULATION: Dementia should be considered a possibility in every hospital patient age 75 and over and can be present in younger patients as well. People with dementia usually come into a hospital for treatment of their other medical conditions, although some come in because of complications of their dementia. Of older people with dementia, 30% also had coronary artery disease; 28% congestive heart failure (CHF); 21% diabetes; and 17% chronic obstructive pulmonary disease (COPD). [i]

BEST PRACTICES: There are four basic approaches to increase recognition of dementia in older hospital patients. The **first** approach is to ask the person and family if the person has "severe memory problems" [ii] and **second**, if a doctor has ever said that the person has Alzheimer's disease or dementia. [iii] The easiest way to do this is to add the items "severe memory problems," "Alzheimer's disease," and "dementia" to the list of diseases and conditions patients and families are routinely asked about on intake forms and in intake interviews.

Two instruments can be used alert staff to the possibility of dementia. The approaches exemplified in these instruments identify "triggers" that indicate a possible problem and need for further assessment. It should be noted that reliability for these instruments has not been established. Hospitals should consider which approach(es) will work best within their existing admission procedures. A combination of approaches may be most effective.

When no prior diagnosis of dementia is reported:

1. *Family Questionnaire:* A family member or friend who accompanies the patient to the hospital can be handed a print copy of the 7-item Family Questionnaire. This questionnaire is intended to identify memory problems that interfere with day to day activities – a hallmark sign of possible dementia. As an alternative to the print questionnaire, the intake interviewer or other hospital staff can ask the family member or friend the seven questions. Responses can be scored by staff.

2. *Patient Behavior Triggers for Clinical Staff:* This tool includes signs and symptoms that suggest the need to consider dementia. The intake interviewer and other hospital staff can be asked to record or report signs and symptoms of possible dementia.[iv]

Note: At the time of hospital intake, it is very difficult to differentiate dementia and delirium, and many older patients with dementia also have delirium.[vii] None of the approaches above rule out delirium. Further assessment is needed for this purpose.

MORE ON THE TOPIC:

i   Bynum JPW, Rabins PV, Weller W, et al. (2004). The relationship between a dementia diagnosis, chronic illness, Medicare expenditures, and hospital use. *Journal of the American Geriatrics Society*, 52:187-194.

ii   This item, 'severe memory problems,' is one of 18 conditions listed in Kaiser Permanente's health risk assessment instrument for Medicare beneficiaries.

iii This question comes from the Medicare Current Beneficiary Survey.

iv   This approach was used in an emergency room study: Mion LC, Palmer RM, Anetzberger GJ, et al. (2001) Establishing a case-finding and referral system for at-risk older individuals in the emergency department setting: the SIGNET model. *Journal of the American Geriatrics Society*, 49:1379-1386.

v   This questionnaire is adapted for the hospital setting from an instrument developed for the Chronic Care Networks for Alzheimer's Disease project, a joint project of the Alzheimer's Association and the National Chronic Care Consortium. The problems in the everyday activities it asks about are widely accepted signs of possible dementia. Costa PT, Williams TF, Albert MS, et al. (1996) *Recognition and Initial Assessment of Alzheimer's Disease and Related Dementias*, USDHHS, Agency for Health Care Policy and Research, Rockville, MD.

vi   These items were adapted for the hospital setting from "triggers" noted in Costa et. al. (1996) (above) and a similar tool developed for the Chronic Care Networks for Alzheimer's Disease project, a joint project of the Alzheimer's Association and the National Chronic Care Consortium.

vii Fick D, and Foreman M. (2000). Consequences of not recognizing delirium superimposed on dementia in hospitalized elderly individuals. *Journal of Gerontological Nursing*, 26:130-140.

FIGURE 12.1 *Try This: Recognition of Dementia in Hospitalized Older Adults.*

BEST TOOLS:

Family Questionnaire [v]

Please answer the following questions. This information will help us provide better care for your family member or friend. Thinking back over the past six months, before hospitalization, would you say your family member or friend has had problems with any of the following? Please circle the answer.

1. Repeating or asking the same thing over and over?	Not at all	Sometimes	Frequently	N/A
2. Forgetting appointments, family occasions, holidays?	Not at all	Sometimes	Frequently	N/A
3. Writing checks, paying bills, balancing the checkbook?	Not at all	Sometimes	Frequently	N/A
4. Shopping independently for clothing or groceries?	Not at all	Sometimes	Frequently	N/A
5. Taking medications according to instructions?	Not at all	Sometimes	Frequently	N/A
6. Getting lost while walking or driving in familiar places?	Not at all	Sometimes	Frequently	N/A
7. Making decisions that arise in everyday living?	Not at all	Sometimes	Frequently	N/A

Relationship to patient _____ *(spouse, son, daughter, brother, sister, grandchild, friend, etc.)*
This information will be given to the patient's doctor and nurse. Thank you for your help.

How to Use the Family Questionnaire:
If a family member or friend is with the patient, tell the patient you have a few questions for his or her family member or friend that will help you find out if the patient has trouble remembering or thinking clearly. Explain that this information may not come to the hospital's attention unless you ask about it and that the information will help you take better care of the patient. Show the questionnaire to the patient if he or she asks to see it. Be sure the patient consents, then hand the questionnaire to the family member or friend. Once it is completed, score the questionnaire, and attach it to the patient's chart.

Scoring:

Not at all or N/A	= 0	
Sometimes	= 1	
Frequently	= 2	**Total Score:** _____

Score Interpretation: *A score of 3 or more should prompt further assessment. A score of 3-6 indicates possible dementia. A score of 7-10 indicates probable dementia.*

Patient Behavior Triggers for Clinical Staff [vi]

Individuals with undiagnosed dementia may exhibit behaviors or symptoms that offer a clue to the presence of dementia, for example, if the patient:

• Seems disoriented
• Is a *"poor historian"*
• Defers to a family member to answer questions directed to the patient
• Repeatedly and apparently unintentionally fails to follow instructions
• Has difficulty finding the right words or uses inappropriate or incomprehensible words
• Has difficulty following conversations

How to Use the Patient Behavior Triggers:
These triggers can be used on a laminated card or other convenient form to remind staff of signs and symptoms that indicate a need for dementia assessment.

When the results of any of these approaches indicate possible dementia, further assessment is needed to measure the level of cognitive impairment and identify delirium, depression, and other conditions that can cause of cognitive impairment. For assessment instruments that are useful for this purpose, see *Try This: Mini Mental State Examination* (MMSE); *Try This: Confusion Assessment Method* (CAM); *Try This: Brief Evaluation of Executive Dysfunction*; and *Try This: Geriatric Depression Screening* (GDS), all available at www.hartfordign.org

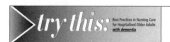

A series provided by The Hartford Institute for Geriatric Nursing and the Alzheimer's Association **www.hartfordign.org**	alzheimer's ℜ association

have depressed mood (Grossberg & Desai, 2003). Depression worsens the prognosis in dementia (Barak & Eisenberg, 2002). On the other hand, people with dementia and depression are known to respond well to treatment of their depression (Eccles, Clarke, Livingston, Freemantle, & Mason, 1998).

This issue from the original *Try This* series (Kurlowicz, 1999) recommends the use of the Geriatric Depression Scale (GDS) (Yesavage, Brink, Rose, Lum, Huang, & Adey, et al., 1983) for assessment of depression in people with dementia. It should be noted, however, that the GDS is a screening tool, and further evaluation by mental health professionals is necessary if the test indicates depressive symptoms.

TRY THIS: BEST PRACTICES IN NURSING CARE FOR HOSPITALIZED OLDER ADULTS WITH DEMENTIA

In addition to *Try This: Recognition of Dementia in Hospitalized Older Adults,* five additional issues for the new *Try This* series were completed by Summer 2004. These five issues, all of which focus on care for hospitalized older adults with dementia, are described below. Following this section is a description of six additional issues that are forthcoming.

Try This: Avoiding Restraints in Patients with Dementia

Older adults with dementia have the highest risk of being restrained. Restraints include posey vests, limb restraints, waist restraint, and full-length siderails. Memory disorder, decreased comprehension, and impaired judgment result in decreased safety awareness, predisposing the demented person to falls and injuries. This is the most commonly cited reason for restraint use. Restraints are also often used to prevent wandering and to prevent patients from interfering with treatment such as feeding tubes and intravenous lines (Strumpf, Robinson, Wagner, & Evans, 1998).

Try This: Avoiding Restraints in Patients with Dementia (Cotter & Evans, 2003) provides alternatives to restraint use, including:

- Assessment for causes of confusion and behavior
- Communication techniques that promote a sense of patient well being
- Equipment and environmental modification, including the use of low beds and bedside mats as alternatives to full siderails

- Involvement of family in care
- Organizational changes, including consistent assignment of staff to promote follow-through of care and patient security

Best practices support individualized care based on diligent assessment, provided by an interdisciplinary team of nurses, physicians, and rehabilitation staff (Capezuti, Talerico, Cochran, Becker, Strumpf, & Evans, 1999). See Figure 12.2 for the *Try This: Avoiding Restraints in Patients with Dementia.*

Try This: Assessing Pain in Persons with Dementia

Cognitively impaired older adults may fail to interpret sensations as painful, are often unable to recall their pain, and may not be able to describe their pain (Horgas & Tsai, 1998). As a result, they are often undertreated for pain. In *Try This: Assessing Pain in Persons with Dementia,* Horgas (2003) recommends that patients with cognitive loss be assessed upon admission to the hospital and again periodically, using a standardized assessment tool such as the Verbal Descriptor Scale (Herr, 2002). This tool requires that the patient have the cognitive ability to describe his or her present pain intensity (e.g., "no pain" to "worst pain" imaginable).

Horgas (2003) further advises that, for the patient with dementia, the clinician utilize the Checklist for Nonverbal Pain Behavior (Feldt, 2000) This tool measures pain by observing patient expressions, including vocal complaints, facial grimaces, bracing, restlessness, and rubbing (Feldt, 2000). The presence of any of the behavioral indicators may be indicative of pain and warrants further investigation, treatment, and monitoring. If pain is suspected, a time-limited trial of a mild analgesic should be initiated. The patient should then be observed closely for changes in expression, behavior, and movement consistent with alleviation of pain (Kovatch, Weissman, Griffie, Matson, & Muchka, 1999; Weiner & Hanlon, 2001). See Figure 12.3 for *Try This: Assessing Pain in Persons with Dementia.*

Try This: Wandering in the Hospitalized Older Adult

Hospital patients with dementia are at risk for wandering and getting lost, either in or outside the hospital. Once lost, they are in danger of injury and even death from falls, accidents, and exposure. The acute medical conditions that initially brought these patients to the hospital compound the likelihood of serious negative outcomes from wandering

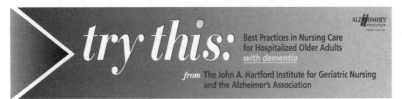

Volume 1, Number 2, Summer 2003   Series Editor: Cora Zembrzuski, APRN, MSN, CS, PhD (c)

Avoiding Restraints In Patients with Dementia

By: Valerie T. Cotter, MSN, CRNP and Lois K. Evans, DNSc, RN, FAAN

WHY: Use of physical restraints in older adults is associated with poor outcomes: functional decline, decreased peripheral circulation, cardiovascular stress, incontinence, muscle atrophy, pressure ulcers, infections, agitation, social isolation, psychiatric morbidity, serious injuries and death. Older adults with dementia have the highest risk of all patients for being restrained when hospitalized. Impaired memory, judgment, and comprehension contribute to the difficulty these patients have in adapting to the hospital. Patients may feel 'lost' and afraid, and try to escape or 'resist' care, yet language deficits associated with dementia limit their ability to clearly express these concerns. Brain damage associated with dementia also places these patients at risk for delirium or acute confusional state, further increasing disorientation and confusion.

TARGET POPULATION: Older adults admitted directly from home, nursing home or other non-hospital setting. At particular risk for restraint use are patients whose behavior (agitation, confusion, exiting the bed unassisted) is judged to be 'unsafe', i.e., contributing to falls and interfering with treatment and medical devices.

BEST PRACTICE: Best practice supports individualized care that permits **nursing the person safely** and without physical or chemical restraint. There is no single instrument to assess the meaning of behavioral communication in hospitalized older adults with dementia. Knowledge about the patient's usual behavior and function is critical to individualizing care. Standardized screening of cognition and to detect delirium should be done at admission and periodically (See *Try This*: Mini Mental State Exam; Confusion Assessment Method).

ASSESS COMMUNICATION AND BASELINE BEHAVIORS; ASSESS RESTRAINT RISK

▸ **Assess the message in the patient's behavior**
  • **Ask the patient what she or he needs:** Many patients with dementia can still communicate needs.

▸ Consult knowledgeable others: Ascertain the patient's personal and medical history, typical communication style, behavior, daily routines, and abilities.

▸ **Assess for unmet needs and behavioral changes:**
  • Use increased confusion and agitation to trigger assessment for changes in the patient's health status.
  • Assess for hunger, fatigue, sleep deprivation, pain, need to urinate or defecate, infection, obstruction, fear or hallucinations. Listen "beyond the words" to understand the emotions behind what the patient is trying to communicate.

▸ **Use standardized screening instruments on admission and periodically; Use any change from baseline to trigger further assessment:** Screen for cognitive function (e.g., Mini Mental State Exam-MMSE), delirium (e.g., Confusion Assessment Method-CAM), and mobility and transfer performance (ADLs). See The Hartford Institute for Geriatric Nursing website at hartford.ign@nyu.edu

▸ **Assess behavior that places a patient at risk for restraint use:**
  • Fall risk; *restraints do not prevent falls or fall-related injuries*
  • Interference with treatment devices (feeding tubes, intravenous lines, sensors and monitors, urinary catheters, dressings, oxygen catheters or mask, ventilators)
  • Agitation, restlessness, bed exits

USEFUL INTERVENTIONS TO PREVENT AND RESPOND TO PATIENT BEHAVIORS

Match specific interventions to the individual patient and his/her needs

▸ *Communicate clearly, slowly, calmly:* Face the patient; always call the patient by the preferred name; use gestures; relax and smile

▸ <u>Remove bedside rails or use only half rails; remove restraints</u>

FIGURE 12.2 *Try This: Avoiding Restraints in Persons with Dementia.*

▸ **Understand the patient's reason for attempting bed exit:** Most often, it is a <u>need to toilet</u>. Anticipate and meet needs by individualized elimination routine based on the patient's history.

▸ **Attend to bed safety:** Lower height, alarms, bed-boundary markers, trapeze or transfer enabler.
  • **Remember, an alarm system is merely *an alert* for a potential emergency.**
  • **Identify all patients on each shift that have bed alarms**

▸ **Attend to chair and wheelchair safety:** Use portable chair alarms

▸ **Protect against falls and injuries**
  • Provide night light in bathroom
  • Preserve function with daily weight-bearing, comfortable seating, ambulation devices at the bedside
  • Provide non-skid slippers
  • Place fall risk "alert" on the bed or door frame
  • Be especially alert at change of shift times

▸ **Modify the immediate environment:**
  • Reduce excessive noise and activity (TV off unless patient requests)
  • Provide for interaction with and visualization of and by others
  • Provide appropriate light levels
  • Remove confusing art or other objects

▸ **Provide surveillance:** Move patient closer to nursing station or to a room with a window to the hallway; use monitors

▸ **Reassess need for invasive treatment devices**
  • **Use the Least Invasive Method to Deliver Care**
  • **Repeatedly use verbal explanation, guided exploration and a mirror:** Help the patient understand what is in place and why
  • **Provide comfort care to the site:** Oral/nasal care, anchoring of tubing
  • **Use camouflage:** Clothing or elastic sleeves, temporary air splint
  • **Provide diversionary activities:** Something to hold and squeeze; favorite music in a headset
  • **Discontinue invasive treatments as early as possible**

▸ **Provide for 'familiarity':** Encourage use of family photographs, favorite personal mementos, audiotapes of family members. Assign the same staff to the extent possible.

▸ **Encourage family and familiar others to participate in care:** Frequent visiting, ADL assistance, and remaining at the bedside around the clock for 1-2 days post admission and/or during the evening

▸ Strive for consistency of personnel, normal function and usual routines, e.g., toileting, eating, and personal hygiene care

ORGANIZATIONAL STRUCTURE TO SUPPORT RESTRAINT-FREE CARE

▸ Establish a Restraint Reduction committee

▸ Review the organization's mission statement, policies; assure committed leadership

▸ Use geriatric advanced practice nurses, physicians, and interdisciplinary team consultation for complex patient presentations

▸ Provide staff education; consistent staff assignment; access to supportive equipment; technology to support reliable admission data and communication of care strategies

▸ Review pain evaluation and treatment protocols

▸ Test patient interventions through continuous quality improvement (CQI)

REFERENCES:

Capezuti, E., Talerico, K.A., Cochran, I., Becker, H., Strumpf, N., & Evans, L. (1999). Individualized interventions to prevent bed-related falls and reduce siderail use. *Journal of Gerontological Nursing*, 25(11), 26-34.

DeProspero, P., & Bocchino, N.L. (1999). Restraint-free care: Is it possible? *American Journal of Nursing*, 99(10), 26-33.

Strumpf, N.E., Robinson, J.P., Wagner, J.S., & Evans, L.K. (1998). *Restraint-free care*, New York: Springer.

Sullivan-Marx, E.M. (2001). Achieving restraint-free care of acutely confused older adults. *Journal of Gerontological Nursing*, 27(4), 56-61.

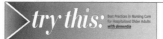

A series provided by
The Hartford Institute for Geriatric Nursing
and the Alzheimer's Association
www.hartfordign.org

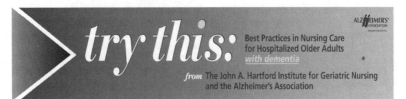

Volume 1, Number 2, Fall 2003   Series Editor: Cora Zembrzuski, APRN, MSN, CS, PhD (cand.)

Assessing Pain in Persons with Dementia

Ann L. Horgas, RN PhD

WHY: There is no evidence that persons with dementia physiologically experience less pain than do other older adults. Rather than being less sensitive to pain, cognitively-impaired elders may fail to interpret sensations as painful, are often less able to recall their pain, and may not be able to verbally communicate it to their care providers. As such, cognitively impaired older adults are often under-treated for pain (Horgas & Tsai, 1998).

As with all older adults, those with dementia are at risk for multiple sources and types of pain, including chronic pain from conditions such as osteoarthritis and acute pain. Untreated pain in cognitively impaired older adults can delay healing, disturb sleep and activity patterns, reduce functioning, reduce quality of life, and prolong hospitalization.

TARGET POPULATION: Older patients who, because of cognitive impairments, may not be able to be assessed for pain using standardized pain assessment instruments. Thus, beginning with the individual's reentrance into the hospital, whether through planned or emergent entry, interpreting behaviors and assessing pain is essential.

BEST TOOLS: Currently, there are few valid and reliable tools available specifically to measure pain in older adults with dementia. We recommend the following:

▸ Use a standardized tool to assess pain, if possible. Many persons with dementia can respond to pain measures such as the Verbal Descriptor Scale (Herr, 2002; see also *Try This* on pain assessment). This tool measures pain intensity by asking participants to select a word that best describes their present pain (e.g., no pain to worst pain imaginable). This measure has been found to be a reliable and valid measure of pain intensity, and is reported to be the easiest to complete and the most preferred by older adults (Herr & Mobily, 1993).

▸ Use an observational tool to measure the presence of pain in persons with dementia. The *Checklist for Nonverbal Pain Behaviors* (Feldt, 2000) is designed to assess pain behaviors in post-operative patients. This measure has high inter-rater reliability (93% agreement; Kappa = .63 to .82) and is positively associated with self-reports of pain. The presence of a pain indicator is scored as a 1, and the total number of indicators are summed for those occurring at rest, with movement, and overall. The relationship between scores on this tool and pain intensity ratings has not yet been established; i.e., there are no clear cutoff scores to indicate pain severity. Instead, the presence of any of the behavioral indicators listed may be indicative of pain, and warrants further investigation, treatment, and monitoring by the practitioner.

▸ Ask family or usual caregivers as to whether the patient's current behavior (i.e. crying out, restlessness) is different from their customary behavior. This change in behavior may signal pain.

▸ If pain is suspected, consider a time-limited trial of a mild analgesic agent, such as acetaminophen. Thoroughly investigate behavior changes in persons with dementia and, once other causes have been ruled out, initiate a trial of analgesic. Observe closely for changes in expression, behavior, and movement consistent with alleviation of pain (Kovach et al., 1999; Weiner & Hanlon, 2001).

STRENGTHS and LIMIATAIONS: Pain is a subjective experience and there are no definitive, universal tests for pain. For patients with dementia, it is particularly important to know the patient and to consult with family and close contacts.

BARRIERS to PAIN MANAGEMENT in PERSONS with DEMENTIA: There are many barriers to effective pain management in this population. Some common myths are:

(a) pain is a normal part of aging
(b) if a person doesn't say they have pain, they must not be experiencing it, and
(c) that strong analgesics (e.g., opioids) must be avoided in elderly.

A more effective approach to pain management in persons with dementia is to assume that they do have pain if they have conditions and/or medical procedures that are typically associated with pain. That is, take a proactive approach in listening and observing for pain and take steps to alleviate it.

FIGURE 12.3   *Try This: Assessing Pain in Persons with Dementia.*

References

Feldt, K. S. (2000). The checklist of nonverbal pain indicators (CNPI). *Pain Management Nursing*, 1(1), 13-21.

Herr, K. (2002). Chronic pain: Challenges and assessment strategies. *Journal of Gerontological Nursing*, 28 (1), 20-27.

Herr KA, Mobily PR. (1993). Comparison of selected pain assessment tools for use with the elderly. *Applied Nursing Research*. 6, 39-46.

Horgas, A. L., & Tsai, P. F. (1998). Analgesic drug prescription and use in cognitively impaired nursing home residents. *Nursing Research*, 47, 235-242.

Kovach, C., Weissman, D., Griffie, J., Matson, S., & Muchka, S. (1999). Assessment and treatment of discomfort for people with late-stage dementia. *Journal of Pain and Symptom Management*, 18, 412-419.

Weiner, D.K., Hanlon, J.T. (2001). Pain in nursing home residents: Management strategies. *Drugs & Aging*, 18, 13-29.

Date: _____   Patient ID: _____

Hospital Day _____

Checklist of Nonverbal Pain Indicators

(Write a 0 if the behavior was not observed, and a 1 if the behavior occurred even briefly during activity or rest.)	With Movement	Rest
1. Vocal complaints: Non-verbal (Expression of pain, not in words, moans, groans, grunts, cries, gasps, sighs)		
2. Facial Grimaces/Winces (Furrowed brow, narrowed eyes, tightened lips, jaw drop, clenched teeth, distorted expressions).		
3. Bracing (Clutching or holding onto side rails, bed, tray table, or affected area during movement)		
4. Restlessness (Constant or intermittent shifting of position, rocking, intermittent or constant hand motions, inability to keep still)		
5. Rubbing (Massaging affected area)		
(In addition, record Verbal complaints). 6. Vocal complaints: Verbal (Words expressing discomfort or pain, "ouch," "that hurts"; cursing during movement, or exclamations of protest (e.g., stop; that's enough)		
Subtotal Scores		
Total Score		

Feldt, K. S. (1996). Treatment of pain in cognitively impaired versus cognitively intact post hip fractured elders. (Doctoral dissertation, University of Minnesota, 1996). Dissertation Abstracts International, 57-09B, 5574.

Feldt, K.S. (2000). Checklist of Nonverbal Pain Indicators. Pain Management Nursing, 1 (1), 13-21.

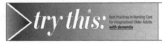

A series provided by
The Hartford Institute for Geriatric Nursing
and the Alzheimer's Association
www.hartfordign.org

REPROGRAPHICS / 190522

and getting lost. Moreover, the strange environment, unfamiliar faces and sounds, and increased confusion due to their acute medical condition, pain, medications, or other treatments may exacerbate pre-existing tendencies to wander. In this *Try This* issue, Silverstein and Flaherty (2004) recommend many approaches nurses and others can use to prevent and manage wandering behaviors: for example, assessment of a patient's risk for wandering, provision of appropriate supervision for the patient; and reduction in environmental triggers for wandering, such as exit signs, suitcases, and street clothes. The authors also recommend that hospitals establish response protocols for the likely event that a patient with dementia will wander and become lost at some time in the future.

See Figure 12.4 for *Try This: Wandering in the Hospitalized Older Adult.*

Try This: Therapeutic Activity Kits

Hospital patients with dementia may have feelings, such as frustration, boredom, loneliness, or anxiety, that they cannot express due to impairments in language, memory, and executive function. Instead they may express these feelings through resistance to personal care, wandering, constant requests for assistance, and repetitive calling out. Unfamiliar surroundings and an overstimulating environment may also provoke patient distress. In this *Try This* issue, Conedera and Mitchell (2004) recommend the use of activity kits to provide cognitive stimulation and make the time the patient spends alone, between staff and family visits, meaningful and less frightening. The issue lists many items that can be included in an activity kit and describes the performance skills required and the therapeutic goals to be achieved with each item.

See Figure 12.5 for *Try This: Therapeutic Activity Kits.*

Try This: Brief Evaluation of Executive Dysfunction: An Essential Refinement in the Assessment of Cognitive Impairment

Executive dysfunction is impairment in cognitive flexibility, concept formation, and self-monitoring, and occurs in all dementias, even when memory impairment is mild (Kennedy & Scalmati, 2002). Executive function is critical for the successful performance of instrumental activities of daily living, such as driving, managing finances, and shopping and should be evaluated when a patient, not thought to have dementia prior to hospitalization, does not return to baseline cognitive function. It is crucial to detect the subtle impairments that may have impacts on the patient's ability to make healthcare decisions and to be discharged safely to home (Kennedy, 2003).

In this *Try This* issue, Kennedy (2003) recommends that the following instruments be used to assess for executive dysfunction:

- Royall's CLOX. The patient is asked to draw a clock set at 1:45, then to copy a clock drawing set at 1:45. The tester evaluates for the following elements: recognizable circle at least one inch in circumference, with all numbers present, in correct symmetrical sequence, with two hands pointing to the correct time. Failure to provide any one of the elements indicates probable impairment.
- The Controlled Oral Word Association Test (Spreen & Benton, 1977). This test asks the patient to list words of three or more letters that begin with the letter "F," "A," and "S." This test evaluates the person's ability to problem solve, sequence, and resist distractions. Persons with intact executive function will produce ten words in each category within one minute.
- The Trailmaking Test, Oral Versions (Ricker & Axelrod, 1994). This test requires the person to count from 1 to 25 and recite 24 letters of the alphabet. The patient is asked to pair numbers and letters, for example, "1-A, 2-B, 3-C," etc., until the digit 13 is reached. The patient is required to sequence items correctly. More than two errors in thirteen pairings is considered impairment.

See Figure 12.6 for the *Try This: Brief Evaluation of Executive Dysfunction.*

FUTURE TOPICS OF *TRY THIS:* BEST PRACTICES IN NURSING CARE FOR HOSPITALIZED OLDER ADULTS WITH DEMENTIA

The following topics are planned for the new *Try This* series in the near future:

- *Communication*—this issue will describe techniques to assist the patient to understand and to be understood.
- *Promoting Family Involvement in Care*—this issue will discuss identification of family members as caregivers and assessment of their desire and ability to be involved in direct care, emotional support, decision-making, and other caregiving functions.

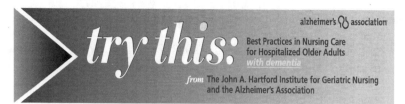

Volume 1, Number 6, Summer 2004   Series Editor: Marie Boltz, APRN, MSN, GNP

Wandering in the Hospitalized Older Adult

By: Nina M. Silverstein, Ph.D., and Gerald Flaherty

WHY: Hospital patients with dementia are at risk for wandering and getting lost either in or outside the hospital. Once lost, they are in danger of injury and even death from falls, accidents, and exposure.[i] The acute medical conditions that initially brought these patients to the hospital compound the likelihood of serious negative outcomes from wandering and getting lost.

Research shows that the majority of older adults with dementia who are ambulatory wander at some time, whether they live at home or in a residential care facility.[ii] The number of patients with dementia who exhibit this behavior in the hospital is not known. Some characteristics of the hospital setting may discourage wandering, but other characteristics of the setting and hospital experience probably promote the behavior. In general, people with dementia wander because they are disoriented, restless, agitated, or anxious; because they are looking for something (e.g., the bathroom, something to eat, or a familiar person or place); or because they think they need to fulfill former obligations, such as work or child care.[iii] As a result of disturbed sleep patterns, they may wander unexpectedly at night. When they are hospitalized, the strange environment, unfamiliar faces and sounds, and increased confusion due to their acute medical condition, pain, medications, or other treatments may exacerbate pre-existing tendencies to wander. For these reasons, even individuals with dementia who do not wander at home or in their residential care facility might wander and get lost in the hospital.

Although many older hospital patients have dementia and are therefore at risk for wandering and getting lost, hospital nurses may not know how to identify this risk. They may also not be aware of approaches they can use to reduce wandering and avoid its potentially dangerous outcomes.

TARGET POPULATION: Older adults with dementia diagnoses and other older adults whose memory loss and other dementia symptoms have not been diagnosed or may not even have been recognized before their hospitalization.

BEST PRACTICE: Best practice in care of hospitalized older adults with dementia involves: 1) identifying risk for wandering, 2) providing appropriate supervision, 3) reducing environmental triggers for wandering, and 4) using individualized nursing interventions to address the causes of wandering behavior.

For hospitals, a lost patient is an emergency. Given the large number of older patients with dementia and the associated risk for wandering, hospitals should have in place protocols for finding lost patients and notifying police and relatives, but many do not.[ii] Hospital nurses can help by advocating with hospital administrators for the development of such protocols.

MORE ON THE TOPIC:

i   Kennedy DB. (1993). Precautions for the physical security of the wandering patient. *Security Journal*, 4(4), 170-176;
      Koester RJ, & Stooksbury DE. (1995). Behavioral profile of possible Alzheimer's patients in Virginia search and rescue incidents.
      Wilderness and Environmental Medicine, 6(1), 34-43.
ii   Silverstein NM, Flaherty G, and Salmons Tobin T. (2002). *Dementia and Wandering Behavior: Concern for the Lost Elder.* New York,
      NY: Springer Publishing Company.
iii   Algase, D.L., (1999). Wandering: A dementia-compromised behavior. *Journal of Gerontologic Nursing*, 25 (9), 10-17.;
      Rader J, Doan J, and Schwab M. (1985). How to decrease wandering, a form of agenda behavior. *Geriatric Nursing*, 6(4):196-199.

FIGURE 12.4   *Try This: Wandering in the Hospitalized Older Adult.*

APPROACHES TO PREVENT/MANAGE WANDERING

Identify risk for wandering

- Be aware of possible dementia; see *Try This: Recognition of Dementia*.
- Assess for memory problems, disorientation, acute confusion, and other mental status changes; see *Try This: Mini Mental State Examination* (MMSE) and *Try This: Confusion Assessment Method* (CAM).
- Ask family members and other caregivers, if any, whether the patient has a history of wandering.

Patients with positive findings from any of the steps above should be considered at risk for wandering and becoming lost in or outside the hospital. The following are suggested approaches to reduce wandering and avoid related injury in this population:

Provide appropriate supervision

- Do not leave the patient alone in the admissions area or waiting for x-rays or other tests.
- Place the patient in a room that allows for maximum staff surveillance; exit paths should intersect with the nurse's station.
- Conduct regular patient checks, especially at shift change.
- Use volunteers, paid "sitters," or specialized staffing as needed.
- Consider different color or patterned hospital gowns for patients at risk of wandering.
- Consider pressure pad alarm sensors on beds and chairs.
- Consider an electronic system using radio frequency transmissions emitted from a wristwatch-like "tag" to monitor patient movement from a central nurses' station.

Reduce environmental triggers for wandering

- Avoid rooms near areas of high traffic or noise.
- Keep stairs, elevators, and other exit cues out of the patient's view.
- Keep suitcases, shoes, and street clothes out of the patient's view.
- Position bed for best visibility and access to the bathroom; use orienting symbols to identify the bathroom (reds are most visible to the aging lens).

Provide individualized nursing interventions to address the causes of wandering

- Ask the family and other caregivers, if any, about the causes of wandering in the past (e.g., restlessness, search for loved ones, trying to "go to work") and specific strategies they have used to reduce wandering (e.g., specific calming, cueing, or redirection strategies).
- Provide a sense of belonging and personal security; reassure the patient that he/she is belongs in the room and is safe there; encourage family and other caregivers to reassure the patient about his/her security in the room.
- Avoid the confusion and anxiety of room changes whenever possible.
- Reduce noise, play soothing music, and use non-glare lighting, all of which may also help decrease agitation that can lead to wandering.
- Encourage movement and exercise; walk with the patient, as appropriate; identify a safe, continuous loop path, if possible.
- Facilitate "failure-free" activities such as sorting harmless objects (i.e., those not ingestible), or viewing albums of familiar photos. See *Try This: Therapeutic Activity Kit*.
- Avoid physical restraints if possible because they increase agitation and patients can be injured as they try to get out of the restraints; see *Try This: Avoiding Restraints in Patients with Dementia*.
- Assess and treat pain that may cause restlessness; see *Try This: Assessing Pain in Persons with Dementia*.
- Secure medical evaluation to identify and treat reversible causes of acute confusion.
- Provide toileting and incontinence care as needed.
- Accommodate bedtime and sleep rituals to prevent insomnia and nighttime wandering.
- Consider a miniature recording device—this can gently address and cue the patient in a familiar voice to remain in place.

Hospital Protocols for Lost Patients

- Encourage hospital administrators to develop and routinely test response protocols for patients who become lost while hospitalized, including timely notification of local police and the patient's relatives.
- Encourage training for security staff about wandering behavior and search and rescue procedures for missing patients with dementia (available from the Alzheimer's Association).
- Encourage hospital administrators to consider the use of procedures to help identify missing patients (e.g., keeping a current photo of the patient on file and keeping an article of the patient's clothing in a sealed plastic bag for canine use).
- Encourage families to register their relative with dementia in the Alzheimer's Association nationwide Safe Return wanderers alert program operated with support of the U.S. Justice Department; look for evidence of patient's registration in Safe Return (bracelet, necklace, key chain, wallet card).

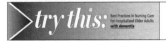

Best Practices in Nursing Care for Hospitalized Older Adults with dementia

A series provided by
The Hartford Institute for Geriatric Nursing
and the Alzheimer's Association
www.hartfordign.org

alzheimer's association

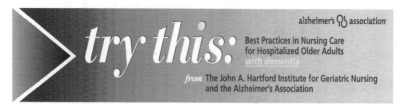

Volume 1, Number 4, Spring 2004   Series Editor: Marie Boltz, APRN, MSN, GNP

Therapeutic Activity Kits
By: Frances Conedera, RN, MS, PMHNP and Laura Mitchell, OTR/L

WHY: Older adults with dementia have feelings that are often difficult to express due to cognitive impairments in language, memory, and executive function. Communicating frustration, boredom, fear, loneliness, anxiety or pain can be expressed as resistance to personal care, wandering, constant requests for assistance, and repetitive calling out. Apraxia, impaired recall, and the attendant anxiety that accompany cognitive loss often impacts the patient's ability to cope with the stress of hospitalization. Caregiver impatience and rushing, being "quizzed" by clinicians and caregivers, unfamiliar surroundings, and an overstimulating environment may also provoke patient distress. Older adults often have periods of intense aloneness in the unfamiliar hospital environment, leading them to seek out companionship and purposeful activity. The use of an activity kit provides an opportunity for cognitive stimulation, and focused and intentional dialogue between caregiver and patient. It can also make the time spent alone, between caregiver and family visits, meaningful and less frightening.

TARGET POPULATION: Hospitalized older adults with suspected or confirmed dementia whether or not they exhibit the behaviors described above, as well as patients with depression and /or limited family contact. Knowledge about the patient's usual behavior and function markedly enhances the ability to individualize care. Standardized screening for cognitive impairment, including dementia, delirium and depression, should be performed upon admission and periodically. (See *Try This*: Mini Mental State Exam, *Try This*: A Brief Evaluation of Executive Dysfunction, *Try This*: Confusion Assessment Method, and *Try This*: Geriatric Depression Scale).

BEST PRACTICES: The evidence suggests that non-pharmacologic methods are effective in improving mood, function and behavior in dementia. An activity kit that is a carefully selected collection of tactile, auditory, and visual items will provide solace, an opportunity for emotional expression, and relief from loneliness and boredom. Added benefits include enhanced cognitive integration, perceptual processing, and neuromuscular strength. The activity kit includes a wide range of items that are commonly used to provide diversion, such as games, audiotapes, and nontoxic art supplies. In addition, items such as pieces of textured fabric, cloth to fold, tools, and key and lock boards, are included for the person with more advanced dementia.

STRENGTHS AND LIMITATIONS: Assessment and appropriate selection of activities is critical to avoid a "quick fix" or overstimulation. The items should reflect/match the patient's preferences, cognitive capacity, and physical abilities. It is crucial to avoid items that infantilize, insult, or threaten the person's self-image. The items listed in this publication are suggestions. Families should be encouraged to individualize contents by providing audiotapes, photo albums, videotapes and activities that the patient enjoys. *All kit items should be provided for the patient to keep, eliminating the need for cleaning between patient use, and infection control concerns.*

ENHANCING USE OF THE KIT: Nursing staff needs to consult with family members and rehabilitation staff regarding the selection of contents, implementation, and evaluation of the activity kit.

References and Resources
Greenwood, D., Loewenthal, D., & Rose, T., (2001). A relational approach to providing care for a person suffering from dementia. *Journal of Advanced Nursing*, 36 (4), 583-590.

Hancock, C., K., (2001). Restraint reduction in acute care. *Journal of Nursing Administration*, 31 (2), 74-77.

Youngstrom, M.J., et al, (2002).Occupational therapy practice framework: domain and process. *American Journal of Occupational Therapy*, 56, 609-639.

Resources for activity materials:
Alimed: HYPERLINK "http://alimed.com" http://alimed.com
Geriatric Resources: HYPERLINK "http://www.geriatric-resources.com" http://www.geriatric-resources.com
Nasco Senior Activities Catalogue, Telephone number: 1-920-563-2446
S&S Primelife, Telephone number: 1-800-243-9232

FIGURE 12.5   *Try This: Therapeutic Activity Kits.*

Suggested Therapeutic Activity Kit Contents

Item	Activity	Performance Skills	Target Areas
Peg Board	Place Pegs in resistive plastic board	Psychosocial Cognitive Motor Vision Sensory	Sense of purpose or relaxation Sequencing, spatial operations, categorization Coordination, crossing midline, ROM, pinch Color discrimination, depth perception, eye/hand coordination Proprioception, light touch
Art supplies (Colored pencils, watercolors, paper, clay)	Drawing, painting, sculpting	Psychosocial Cognitive Motor Vision Sensory	Enjoyment/stimulation, sense of purpose, self expression, or relaxation Attention span, spatial operations Fine motor movement Color discrimination, depth perception, visual perceptual skills Light touch
Wash Cloths	Fold towels/Stacking towels	Psychosocial Cognitive Motor Vision Sensory	Stimulation, sense of purpose or relaxation Sequencing, problem solving, attention span ROM, coordination, bilateral integration, pinch Depth perception Light touch
Fit-a-space puzzle	Assemble & take apart various puzzle pieces/shapes Lace shapes together	Psychosocial Cognitive Motor Vision Sensory	Enjoyment/stimulation, sense of purpose or relaxation Object recognition, attention span, spatial operations Coordination, bilateral integration, visual/motor integration Form constancy, position in space, figure ground Proprioception, light touch
Cones	Stacking Cones	Psychosocial Cognitive Motor Vision Sensory	Enjoyment/stimulation, sense of purpose or relaxation Sequencing, attention span, problem solving Grip, ROM Color discrimination Light touch
PVC Piping (Pipe Tree)	Assemble piping in patterns/shapes	Psychosocial Cognitive Motor Vision Sensory	Enjoyment/stimulation, sense of purpose or relaxation Problem solving, motor planning, sustained attention Pinch, grip, coordination, ROM, bilateral integration Eye/hand coordination, visual perceptual skills Proprioception, light touch
Finger Fidgets	Exercise Fingers with ball	Psychosocial Cognitive Motor Vision Sensory	Enjoyment/stimulation, sense of purpose or relaxation Attention span Pinch, coordination, bilateral integration Color stimulation Proprioception, light touch
Playing Cards	Play Games, sorting, shuffling	Psychosocial Cognitive Motor Vision Sensory	Enjoyment/stimulation Sequencing, memory, picture recognition, attention span, categorization Coordination, bilateral integration, ROM visual motor Figure ground, depth perception, visual memory Light proprioception, touch
CD	Listen to music	Cognitive Psycho-Social Sensory	Arousal/Relaxation Enjoyment/stimulation or relaxation Auditory
Videos	Watch movie	Cognitive Psycho-Social Vision Sensory	Arousal, attention span, orientation, memory Enjoyment/stimulation or relaxation, age appropriate Visual attention Visual, auditory

NOTE: Skills required for each task vary and it is up to the professional to determine which activity is appropriate/ most therapeutic for the patient

Psychosocial= emotional wellbeing

Cognitive = cognitive integration

Vision = perceptual processing

Motor = motor/neuromusculoskeletal skills

Sensory – sensory stimulation

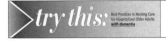 Best Practices in Nursing Care for Hospitalized Older Adults **with dementia**

A series provided by
The Hartford Institute for Geriatric Nursing
and the Alzheimer's Association
www.hartfordign.org

alzheimer's association

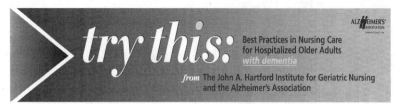

Volume 1, Number 3, Fall 2003   Series Editor: Marie Boltz, RN, MSN, GNP, NHA

Brief Evaluation of Executive Dysfunction:
An Essential Refinement in the Assessment of Cognitive Impairment

By: Gary J. Kennedy MD

WHY: A hospital admission may surface a previously undetected dementia in some older adults. While at home in a familiar environment, patients and family may fail to recognize subtle, slowly progressive cognitive changes. Such changes however, often become apparent when the patient is moved to the unfamiliar setting of the hospital. These are the patients whose family report "my mother was never like this at home."

This *Try This* recommends assessing executive function for older patients not thought to have dementia prior to hospitalization but where the patient, family or staff feel the patient has not returned to baseline cognitive status at the time of discharge. Particularly when the older patient is alert and verbal and **memory is not obviously impaired**, screening for executive dysfunction can be critical to a safe, realistic treatment and discharge plan. Patients who exhibit executive dysfunction should be referred to their primary care provider or to an Aging and Dementia Center.

> **Executive dysfunction defined:** Executive function is an interrelated set of abilities that includes cognitive flexibility, concept formation, and self-monitoring. Assessing executive function can help determine a patient's capacity to execute health care decisions and with discharge planning decisions. With impaired executive dysfunction, instrumental activities of daily living (accounting, shopping, medication management, driving) may be beyond the person's capacity even though memory impairment is mild. The person's capacity to exercise command and self-control, and to direct others to provide care, becomes diminished. Executive dysfunction is one element in the DSM-IV criteria for the diagnosis of dementia and occurs in all dementing diseases.

> NOTE: *Patients with impaired executive function need not have impaired memory.*

TARGET POPULATION: Older patients:

- Not thought to have dementia prior to hospitalization but where the patient, family or staff feel the patient has not returned to baseline cognitive status at the time of discharge.

- For whom other screening (e.g., MMSE, CAM: see *Try This* at www.hartfordign.org) reveals no discernable cause for a cognitive impairment.

- For whom cognitive impairment, observed as alterations in memory, use of language and abstract thinking, and spatial sense, persists even when delirium has been identified and treated or ruled out.

BEST PRACTICES: Few practitioners are familiar with testing for executive function, yet there are valid and reliable instruments. The instruments listed below have good internal consistency, inter-rater reliability and are strongly correlated with the MMSE and with lengthier neuropsychological assessments of executive function:

- Royall's CLOX (clock drawing),

- Controlled Oral Word Association Test, and

- Trailmaking Test, oral version.

FIGURE 12.6   *Try This: Brief Evaluation of Executive Function.*

Further reading:

- Cooney LM, Kennedy GJ, Hawkins KA, Hurme SB. Who can stay at home: Assessing the capacity to choose to live in the community (in press) Archives of Internal Medicine

- Daly S, Sawchuk PJ, Wertenberger DH. Sending the elderly home. Assessing the risk. The Canadian Nurse. 2000; Mar: 27-30.

- Kennedy GJ, Scalmati A: The importance of executive deficits; Assessing the older person's capacity to remain at home: Geriatrics 57:40-41, 2002

- McCullough LB, Molinari V, Workman RH. Implications of impaired executive control functions for patient autonomy and surrogate decision making. J Clinical Ethics. 2001; 12(4):397-405.

- Ricker JH, Axelrod BN. Analysis of an oral paradigm for the trail making test. Assessment 1994;1:47-52

- Royall DR, Cordes JA, Polk M. CLOX: an executive clock drawing task. J Neurol Neurosurg Psychiatry 1998; 64:588-594.

- Royall DR, Cabello M, Polk MJ. Executive dyscontrol: An important factor affecting the level of care received by elderly retirees. J Am Geriatrics Soc 1998;46:1519-1524.

- Spreen FO, Benton AL. Manual of instructions for the Neurosensory Center Comprehensive Examination for Aphasia. Victoria, British Columbia, Canada: University of Victoria. 1977

For complete versions of the CLOX, including a validated Spanish Translation, write to Donald R. Royall MD, Department of Psychiatry, The University of Texas Health Science Center at San Antonio, 7703 Floyd Curl Drive, TX 78284-7792.)

Screening Tests of Executive Function

The following brief screening tests of executive function can be administered in hospital and in the ambulatory setting:

- **Royall's CLOX Clock drawing:** First ask the patient to "Draw me a clock that says 1:45. Set the hands and numbers on the face so that a child could read them." Once the task is complete, draw a clock with a 2 inch diameter, with all the numbers in place, and the hands set at 1:45. Then ask the patient to copy it. An unimpaired person will draw a round figure with the following elements: recognizable circle at least one inch in circumference with all the numbers present and in correct, symmetrical sequence. There will be two hands anchored in the center pointing to the correct time. If any of the above elements are missing the person is possibly impaired. If more than one element is missing the person is probably impaired. Intruded elements such as words or letters indicate impairment. Persons with only executive dysfunction will exhibit errors on the first clock but not the second. Those with both executive function and construction apraxia usually as a result of moderate Alzheimer's disease or stroke will fail both.

- **The Controlled Oral Word Association Test:** With categories beginning with the letter "F", then "A", then "S", the Controlled Oral Word Association Test by Spreen and Benton (1977) requires respondents to fill the category by providing words of 3 or more letters. For example, correct responses to the category cue "F" would include "fish, foul, fact" etc. This test reflects abstract mental operation related to problem solving, sequencing, resisting distractions, intrusions and perseverations. It is considered a "frontal" task as the organization of words by first letter is unfamiliar, and requires conscious, effortful, systematic organization and the filtering of irrelevant information such as natural taxonomic categories. Persons free of executive dysfunction will produce 10 words in each category within one minute.

- **The Trailmaking Test, Oral Version:** (Ricker & Axelrod, 1994) requires the subject to count from 1 to 25 and then recite the 24 letters of the alphabet. For testing the subject is asked to pair numbers and letters e.g. "1-A, 2-B, 3-C, etc." until the digit 13 is reached. This version does not make visual scanning or visually guided motor demands. However, the individual is required to keep the number and letter sequences in working memory so as not to lose place. More than 2 errors in 13 pairings are considered impairment.

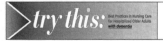

A series provided by
The Hartford Institute for Geriatric Nursing
and the Alzheimer's Association
www.hartfordign.org

REPROGRAPHICS / 187446

- *Meals and Nutrition*—this issue will address the patient's need for assistance during meals, methods of promoting self-care, nutritional needs, and options to promote good nutrition and prevent complications.
- *Decision-making*—this issue will provide techniques for evaluating the patient's ability to make decisions regarding advance directives, discharge planning, and care decisions.
- *Delirium Superimposed on Dementia*—this issue will present a guide for detecting delirium and understanding its underlying causes, including medications, medical problems, depression, and other environmental and emotional factors.
- *Behaviors: restlessness and refusal of care*—this issue will address the meaning behind behaviors that demonstrate patient anxiety and distress and cause stress for nursing staff. Approaches to provide a nonthreatening environment will be given, with the goal of decreasing patient fear, promoting a sense of well-being, and facilitating the delivery of nursing care.

PERTINENT ISSUES FROM THE ORIGINAL *TRY THIS* SERIES

The original *Try This* series was developed to address the assessment of older adults in general, but many of the issues are potentially useful for nurses caring for hospital patients with dementia. The issues described below are particularly pertinent to the prevention and management of common complications of dementia. These documents can be viewed and downloaded from the website of the Hartford Institute, www.hartfordign.org

Try This: Fulmer SPICES: An Overall Assessment Tool for Older Adults

The first issue of the original *Try This* series focuses on the SPICES assessment tool (Wallace & Fulmer, 1998). Each letter in the acronym SPICES stands for an important component of a brief evaluation for older adults, i.e., Sleep disorders, Problems with eating or feeding, Incontinence, Confusion, Evidence of falls, and Skin breakdown. By remembering the word SPICES, nurses can anticipate and assess these commonly occurring problems. Prompt and efficient assessment allows for preventative and therapeutic interventions to be administered early in the development of illness. The SPICES assessment tool was developed and used extensively by nurses in the Geriatric Nurse Resource Project at Yale University Medical Center (Fulmer, 1991a, 1991b).

Try This: Katz Index of Independence in Activities of Daily Living (ADL)

Functional status is the focus of the second issue in the original *Try This* series (Shelkey & Wallace, 1998). The issue highlights the Katz Index of Independence in Activities of Daily Living (1983), more commonly known as the Katz ADL. This instrument assesses functional status by measuring a person's ability to perform six activities of daily living: bathing, dressing, toileting, transferring, continence, and feeding. The Katz ADL instrument has been criticized for its inability to measure small changes in functional status, but it remains one of the most consistently used tools to evaluate the functional status of older adults in multiple settings.

Try This: Elder Abuse and Neglect Assessment

Elder abuse and neglect include the intentional or unintentional abuse and/or neglect, exploitation, or abandonment of an older adult (Fulmer, 2002). Estimates of the prevalence of abuse and neglect of older adults with dementia range from 5% to 12% (Coyne, Reichman, & Berbig, 1993), far exceeding the 1 to 4% rate for all older adults (Lachs, Williams, O'Brien, Hurst, & Horwitz, 1997). However, since abuse and neglect are vastly underreported by older adults and clinical professionals, all these numbers may be considerably higher (Fulmer, 2002).

To improve detection of abuse and neglect, *Try This: Elder Abuse and Neglect Assessment* (Fulmer, 2002) recommends use of of the Elder Assessment Instrument, a 41-item tool that assesses for signs and symptoms consistent with abuse and neglect (for example, physical symptoms without clinical explanation or inconsistent explanation between older adult and caregiver and subjective complaints of abuse or neglect by the older adult) (Fulmer, Street, & Carr, 1984).The instrument is easy to complete and has been used extensively in clinical practice and research (Fulmer, 2002).

Try This: Beers' Criteria for Potentially Inappropriate Medication Use in the Elderly

Excessive and often inappropriate medication use is common in the older population (Morley, 2003). This *Try This* issue points out that nurses' awareness of inappropriate medication use among older adults is essential for preventing adverse effects (Moloney, 2003).

The adapted Beers' Criteria (HCFA Guidelines for Potentially Inappropriate Medications in the Elderly; Beers, 1997) provide a valuable framework to assist in the identification of high-risk medications in the older adult population. These criteria have been successfully used in many settings to detect the use of high-risk medications among older adults, so that actions can be taken to change medications or diminish the risk of adverse effects.

Try This: Caregiver Strain Index (CSI)

As eloquently reported in the book, *The-36 Hour Day* (Mace & Rabins, 2001), dementia caregiving is associated with multiple stressors resulting in depression, grief, fatigue, decreased socialization, development of health problems in the caregiver, and premature institutionalization of the person with dementia. It is essential for nurses to understand the burden of caregiving and to assess caregivers in order to prevent the development or exacerbation of these stress-related problems. This *Try This* issue (Sullivan, 2002) recommends the use of the Caregiver Strain Index (CSI) (Robinson, 1983) for this purpose. The CSI is a thirteen-question instrument that can be administered in a few minutes to identify the level of strain or stress of the caregiver. Items on the instrument focus on difficulties the caregiver may experience in employment, finances, physical health, socialization, and time management. The instrument may be incorporated into the evaluation conducted by a hospital social worker or the psychosocial component of a nursing assessment.

Try This: Predicting Pressure Ulcer Sore Risk

Pressure ulcers occur in 3 to 11% of acute-care patients and 24% of long-term care residents (Ayello, 1999). They are generally caused by prolonged pressure over a bony prominence that results in the compression of the tissue preventing the circulation to the area and resulting in tissue death. Pressure ulcers result in great morbidity for older adults, including pain and perhaps sepsis and death. Older adults with dementia who are unable to articulate the need for repositioning and/or toileting have increased vulnerability for skin breakdown.

Pressure ulcers are entirely preventable. By identifying risk factors for developing them, interventions may be implemented to reduce the risk for the development of these ulcers. In this *Try This* issue, Ayello (1999) recommends the use of the Braden Scale for Predicting Pressure

Sore Risk (Braden, 1997) to detect risk factors leading to the development of pressure ulcers. Once risk factors have been identified, it is essential to implement interventions to reduce the risk and prevent the development and sequelae of pressure sores.

Urinary Incontinence Assessment

Older adults without urinary system pathology experience a decrease in bladder tone and volume capacity that may result in the development of both stress and urge urinary incontinence. Urinary incontinence may also occur as a result of pathological influences on the urinary system, immobility, cognitive impairment, and environmental barriers (Dowling-Castronovo, 2001).

The Agency for Health Care Policy and Research (1996) recommends a bladder diary as the most effective instrument with which to collect information about urinary incontinence. *Try This: Urinary Incontinence Assessment* (Dowling-Castronovo, 2001) provides a sample bladder diary. It also recommends the use of the acronym DIAPPERS for recalling risk factors for the development of urinary incontinence (Resnick, 2003). DIAPPERS stands for *D*elirium, *I*nfection (Urinary Tract), *A*trophic urethritis or vaginitis, *P*harmacology (e.g., diuretics, anticholinergics), *P*sychological disorders (especially depression), *E*ndocrine disorders (e.g., diabetes), *R*estricted mobility (e.g., postoperative), *St*ool impaction. Interventions commonly used to prevent and treat incontinence in a person with dementia include assessment and management of infection, voiding schedules, provision of adequate fluid intake, and environmental cueing to direct the person to the toilet.

Try This: Nutrition and Hydration

Normal and pathological changes of aging, as well as lifestyle and environmental factors, have a profound impact on the nutritional and fluid balance of older adults (Zembrzuski, 2000). It is of utmost importance that the nutritional and fluid status of older adults, especially those with acute and chronic illnesses, be evaluated regularly to ensure prevention and early treatment of potential problems. This *Try This* issue (Zembrzuski, 2000), recommends both the Nutritional Screening Initiative Checklist (NSI) (Dwyer, 1991) and the Hydration Assessment Checklist (Zembrzuski, 1997) for this purpose The NSI may be self-administered by an older person and provides nurses with information on the impact of illness on nutrition and total consumption.The Hydration Assessment Checklist provides a more thorough assessment of the older adult's hydration status, including history, lab results, and intake and output records for three days. It is particularly useful for early detection of dehydration among older adults.

Try This: Fall Risk Assessment

One-third of deaths due to injury in people over 65 are due to falls (Magaziner, Hawkes, Hebel, Zimmerman, Fox, & Dolan, et al. , 2000), and falls are the largest category of adverse incidents in hospitals, with approximately 20% of falls resulting in injury (Kannus Parkkari, Koskinen, Niemi, Palvanen, & Jarvinen, et al., 1999). The risk of falling increases with cognitive impairment due to impaired judgment and lack of safety awareness that occurs in patients with dementia or delirium (Krueger, Brazil, & Lohfeld, 2001). A known diagnosis of dementia is thought to contribute to over 50% of falls in hospitals (Norwalk, Prendergast, Bayles, D'Amico, & Colvin, 2001).

Fall prevention is essential for safe geriatric care and may be best accomplished through a comprehensive falls assessment. There are many fall risk assessments (Hollinger & Patterson, 1992; Tideiksaar, 1996; Tinnetti & Speechley, 1989). This *Try This* issue (Farmer, 2000) recommends the Fall Assessment Tool (Hollinger & Patterson, 1992).

Fall risk assessments should be administered on admission to the hospital and repeatedly administered if a change in health status occurs, or during intervals specified by the facility or agency policy. If a hospitalized patient falls, the nurse should conduct a comprehensive evaluation to assess the factors contributing to the fall and revise the plan of care as indicated (Resnick, 2003).

IMPLICATIONS FOR FUTURE PRACTICE

The Alzheimer's Association and Hartford Institute are committed to the increased distribution of *Try This: Best Practices in Nursing Care for Hospitalized Older Adults with Dementia* to the whole spectrum of hospital practice areas, including emergency and critical care settings. Both the Alzheimer's Association and the Hartford Institute provide ongoing education on *Try This* tools at national conferences and through their respective Web sites and publications. In addition, diverse vehicles of dissemination, including electronic formats, are planned. The goal is to provide easily accessible information in a variety of formats.

Try This instruments can be linked to evidence-based protocols in an electronic documentation system that is efficient and serves to reinforce knowledge of best practices. The NICHE (Nurses Improving the Care of Health System Elders) program, run by the Hartford Institute, works with hospitals to develop clinical expertise, culture change that values gerontologic care, and operational practices that support humane and competent care for the person with dementia. The Hartford Institute plans to support hospitals' efforts to embed the use of *Try This* tools into various nursing care models, including ACE units (specialized hospital units dedicated to the care of acutely ill older adults) and Geriatric Resource Nurse programs (role enhancement for hospital nurses through specialized education in gerontologic nursing).

Easily accessible, the *Try This* series presents an excellent opportunity for direct intervention. Either through in-service training and discussion or individual reference, *Try This* gives nurses one more useful strategy to add to their repertoire.

REFERENCES

Agency for Health Care Policy and Research. (1996). *Urinary incontinence in adults: Acute and chronic management: Clinical practice guideline #2.* AHCPR Publication Number 96–0682, March.

Armstrong-Esther, C., Browne, K., & McAffee, J. (1999). Investigation into nursing staff knowledge and attitudes to dementia. *International Journal of Psychiatric Nursing Research, 4,* 489–487.

Ayello, E. (1999). Predicting pressure ulcer sore risk. *Try this: Best Practices in Nursing Care to Older Adults, 5.* New York: The Hartford Institute for Geriatric Nursing, New York University, Division of Nursing.

Barak, Y., & Eisenberg, D. (2002). Suicide amongst Alzheimer's disease patients: a 10-year survey. *Dementia and Geriatric Cognitive Disorders, 14,* 101–103.

Beers, M. H. (1997). Explicit criteria for determining potentially inappropriate medication use by the elderly. *Archives of Internal Medicine 157,* 1531–1536.

Braden, B. J. (1997). Risk assessment in pressure ulcer prevention. In D. Krasner and D. Kane (Eds.), *Chronic wound care: A clinical source book for healthcare professionals.* (2nd ed.). Health Management Publication: Wayne, PA.

Capezuti, E., Talerico, K., Cochran, I., Becker, H., Strumpf, N., & Evans, L. (1999). Individualized interventions to prevent bed-related falls and reduce side rail use. *Journal of Gerontological Nursing, 25*(11), 26–34.

Conedera, F., & Mitchell, L., (2004). Therapeutic Activity Kits. *Try This: Best practices in nursing care for hospitalized older adults with dementia, 4.* New York: The Hartford Institute for Geriatric Nursing, New York University, Division of Nursing.

Cotter, V., & Evans, L. (2003). Avoiding restraints in patients with dementia. *Try this: Best practices in nursing care for hospitalized older adults with dementia, 2.* New York: The Hartford Institute for Geriatric Nursing, New York University, Division of Nursing.

Coyne, A. C., Reichman,W. E., & Berbig, L.J. (1993). The relationship between dementia and elder abuse. *American Journal of Psychiatry, 150,* 643–646.

Dowling-Castronova, A. (2001). Urinary incontinence assessment. *Try this: Best practices in nursing care to older adults, 11.* New York: The Hartford Institute for Geriatric Nursing, New York University, Division of Nursing.

Dwyer, J. T. (1991). *Screening older American's nutritional health: Current practices and future responsibilities.* Washington, DC: Nutritional Screening Institute.

Eccles, M., Clarke, J., Livingston, M., Freemantle, N., & Mason, J. (1998). North of England evidence-based guidelines development project: guideline for the primary care management of dementia. *British Medical Journal, 317,* 802–808.

Eriksson, C., & Saveman, B-I. (2002). Nurses' experiences of abusive /nonabusive caring for demented patients in acute care settings. *Scandinavian Journal of Caring Sciences, 16,* 79–85.

Farmer, B. C. (2000). Fall Risk Assessment. *Try this: Best practices in nursing care to older adults, 8.* New York: The Hartford Institute for Geriatric Nursing, New York University, Division of Nursing.

Feldt, K. S. (2000). The checklist of nonverbal pain indicators (CPNI). *Pain Management Nursing, 1*(1), 13–21.

Fick, D., Agostini, J., & Inouye, S. (2002). Delirium superimposed on dementia: A systematic review. *Journal of the American Geriatrics Society, 50,* 1723–1732.

Folstein, M., Folstein, S. E., & McHugh, P. R. (1975). "Mini-mental state" a practical method for grading the cognitive state of patients for the clinician. *Journal of Psychiatric Research, 12*(3), 189–198.

Fulmer, T. (1991a). The geriatric nurse specialist role: a new model. *Nursing Management, 22*(3), 91–93.

Fulmer, T. (1991b). Grow your own experts in hospital elder care. *Geriatric Nursing, March/April,* 64–66.

Fulmer, T. (2002). Elder abuse and neglect assessment. *Try this: Best practices in nursing care to older adults, 15*(v2). New York: The Hartford Institute for Geriatric Nursing, New York University, Division of Nursing.

Fulmer, T., Street, S., & Carr, K. (1984). Abuse of the elderly: screening and detection. *Journal of Emergency Nursing, 10*(3), 131–140.

Grossberg, G., & Desai, A. (2003). Management of Alzheimer's disease. *Journal of Gerontology, Biological Sciences and Medical Sciences, 58,* M331–M353.

Hendrie, H. C. (1998). Epidemiology of dementia and Alzheimer's disease. *American Journal of Geriatric Psychiatry, 6.* (2 suppl1), S3–S18.

Herr, K. A. (2002). Chronic pain: Challenges and assessment strategies. *Journal of Gerontological Nursing, 28*(10), 20–7.

Hollinger, L., & Patterson, R. (1992) A fall prevention program for the acute care setting. In S. G. Funk, E. M. Tornquist, M. T. Chanpagne, & R. A. Wiese (Eds.) Key aspects of elder care: Managing falls, incontinence, and cognitive impairment. New York, NY: Springer Publishing Co., Inc.

Horgas, A., (2003) Assessing pain in persons with dementia. *Try this: Best practices in nursing care for hospitalized older adults with dementia, 2.* New York: The Hartford Institute for Geriatric Nursing, New York University, Division of Nursing.

Horgas, A., Wahl, H.W., & Baltes, M. M (1996). Dependency in later life. In L. Carstensen, B. Edelstein, & L. Dornbrand (Eds.), *The practical handbook of clinical gerontology* (pp. 54–75). Thousand Oaks, CA: Sage.

Horgas, A., & Tsai, P. F. (1998). Analgesic drug prescription and use in cognitively impaired nursing home residents. *Nursing Research, 47,* 235–242.

Inouye, S. (1998). Delirium in hospitalized older patients. *Clinics in Geriatric Medicine,* November.

Inouye, S., Van Dyck, C., Alessi, C., Balkin, S., Siegal, A., & Horwitz, R. (1990). Clarifying confusion: the confusion assessment method. *Annals of Internal Medicine, 113*(12), 941–948.

Kannus, P., Parkkari, J., Koskinen, S., Niemi, S., Palvanen, M., & Jarvinen, M., et al. (1999). Fall induced injuries and deaths among older adults. *Journal of the American Medical Association, 189,* 1895–1899.

Katz, S. (1983). Assessing self-maintenance: Activities of daily living, mobility and instrumental activities of daily living. *Journal of the American Geriatrics Society, 31*(12), 721–726.

Kennedy, G. (2003). Brief evaluation of executive dysfunction: An essential refinement in the assessment of cognitive impairment. *Try this: Best practices in nursing care for hospitalized older adults with dementia, 3.* New York: The Hartford Institute for Geriatric Nursing, New York University, Division of Nursing.

Kennedy, G., & Scalmati, A. (2002). The importance of executive deficits: Assessing the older person's capacity to remain at home. *Geriatrics, 57,* 40–41.

Kovach, C., Weissman, D., Griffie, J., Matson, S., & Muchka, S. (1999). Assessment and treatment of discomfort for people with late-stage dementia. *Journal of Pain and Symptom Management, 18,* 412–419.

Krueger, P., Brazil, K., & Lohfeld, L. (2001). Risk factors for falls and injuries on a long-term facility in Ontario. *Canadian Journal of Public Health, 92,* 117–120.

Kurlowicz, L. (1999). The Geriatric Depression Scale. *Try this: Best practices in nursing care to older adults, 4.* New York: The Hartford Institute for Geriatric Nursing, New York University, Division of Nursing.

Kurlowicz, L., & Wallace, M. (1999). The Mini Mental State Examination (MMSE). *Try this: Best practices in nursing care to older adults, 3.* New York: The Hartford Institute for Geriatric Nursing, New York University, Division of Nursing.

Lachs, M. S., Williams, C., O'Brien, S., Hurst, L., & Horwitz, R.(1997). Risk factors for reported elder abuse and neglect: A nine year observational cohort study. *Gerontologist, 37,* 469–474.

Leon, J., Cheng, C. K., & Neumann, P. J. (1998). Alzheimer's disease care: cost and potential savings. *Health Affairs, 17*, 206–216.

Mace, N. L., & Rabins, P. V. (2001). *The 36-hour day: A family guide to caring for persons with Alzheimer disease, related dementing illnesses, and memory loss in later life.* New York: Warner Books.

Magaziner, J., Hawkes, W., Hebel, R., Zimmerman, S., Fox, K., & Dolan, M., et al. (2000). Recovery from hip fracture in eight areas of function. *Journal of Gerontology Medical Sciences, 55A(9),* 498–507.

Mezey, M., & Maslow, K., (2004). Recognition of Dementia in Hospitalized Older Adults. *Try this: Best practices in nursing care for hospitalized older adults with dementia, 5.* New York: The Hartford Institute for Geriatric Nursing, New York University, Division of Nursing.

Moloney, S L. (2003). Beers' criteria for potentially inappropriate medication use in the elderly. *Try this: Best practices in nursing care to older adults, 16.* New York: The Hartford Institute for Geriatric Nursing, New York University, Division of Nursing.

Morley, J. (2003). Hot topics in geriatrics (Editorial). *Journal of Gerontology Medical Sciences, 58A,* 30–36.

Norberg, A. (2001). Communication with people suffering from severe dementia. In M. Clinton and S. Nelson (Eds.), *Advanced practice in mental health nursing,* London: Blackwell Science, 18–72.

Norwalk, M., Prendergast, J., Bayles, C., D'Amico, F., & Colvin, G. (2001). A randomized trial of exercise programs among older individuals living in two long term care facilities: The Falls Free program. *Journal of the American Geriatrics Society, 49,* 859–865.

Resnick, B. (2003) Preventing falls in acute care. In M. Mezey, T. Fulmer, I. Abraham (Eds.), *Geriatric nursing protocols for best practice* (2nd ed.), (pp. 141–164). New York: Springer.

Ricker, J. H., & Axelrod, B. N. (1994). Analysis of an oral paradigm for the trail making test. *Assessment, 1,* 47–52.

Robinson, B. (1983). Validation of a Caregiver Strain Index. *Journal of Gerontology. 38,* 344–348.

Shelkey, M., & Wallace, M. (1998). Katz Index of Independence in Activities of Daily Living. *Try this: Best practices in nursing care to older adults, 2.* New York: The Hartford Institute for Geriatric Nursing, New York University, Division of Nursing.

Silverstein, N. M., & Flaherty, G. (2004). Wandering in the Hospitalized Older Adult. *Try this: Best practices in nursing care for hospitalized older adults with dementia, 6.* New York: The Hartford Institute for Geriatric Nursing, New York University, Division of Nursing.

Spreen, F. O., & Benton, A.L., (1977). Manual of instructions for the Neurosensory Center Comprehensive Examination for Aphasia. Victoria, British Columbia, Canada: University of Victoria.

Strumpf, N. E., Robinson, J. P., Wagner, J. S., & Evans, L. K. (1998). *Restraint-free care.* New York: Springer.

Sullivan, T. M. (2002). Caregiver Strain Index (CSI). *Try this: Best practices in nursing care to older adults, 14.* New York: The Hartford Institute for Geriatric Nursing, New York University, Division of Nursing.

Tideiksaar, R. (1996). Preventing falls: How to identify risk factors, reduce complications. *Geriatrics, 5*(2), 43–46, 49–53.

Tinnetti, M., & Speechley, M. (1989). Prevention of falls among the elderly. *New England Journal of Medicine, 320,* 1055–1059.

Volicer, L., & Hurley, A. C. (1997. Comorbidity in Alzheimer's disease. *Journal of Mental Health & Aging, 3,* 5–17.

Wallace, M., & Fulmer, T. (1998). FULMER SPICES: An overall assessment tool of older adults. *Try this: Best practices in nursing care to older adults, 1.* New York: The Hartford Institute for Geriatric Nursing, New York University, Division of Nursing.

Waszynski, C. M. (2001). Confusion Assessment Method (CAM). *Try this: Best practices in nursing care to older adults, 13.* New York: The Hartford Institute for Geriatric Nursing, New York University, Division of Nursing.

Weiner, D. K., & Hanlon, J. T. (2001). Pain in nursing home residents: Management strategies. *Drugs & Aging, 18,* 13–19.

Yesavage, J. A., Brink, T. L., Rose, T. L., Lum, O., Huang, V., & Adey, M., et al. (1983). Development and validation of a geriatric depression screening scale: A preliminary report. *Journal of Psychiatric Research, 17,* 37–49.

Zembrzuski, C. (1997). A three-dimensional approach to hydration of elders: Adminstration, clinical staff, and inservice education. *Geriatric Nursing, 18*(1), 20–26.

Zembrzuski, C. (2000). Nutrition & hydration. *Try this: Best practices in nursing care to older adults, 9.* New York: The Hartford Institute for Geriatric Nursing, New York University, Division of Nursing.

CHAPTER THIRTEEN

Alzheimer's Association New York City Chapter

Strategies for Improving Hospital Care

Jed A. Levine and Jean Marks

Alzheimer's Association staffs interact extensively with persons with Alzheimer's disease and other dementias and their families and, as a result, are painfully aware of problems these individuals face. Over the years, staff of the New York City Chapter has heard many stories about problems with hospital care. To begin to address this issue, the Chapter was an important catalyst in a multiyear project that led to the creation of a specialized acute care unit for patients with Alzheimer's and other dementias at Cabrini Medical Center. Chapter 11 describes the acute care unit. This chapter describes the New York City Chapter's reasons for participating in the Cabrini project, the Chapter's role in the planning process, and other projects that have evolved from the Chapter's working partnership with Cabrini Medical Center. Lessons from the New York City Chapter's experience and strategies that may be useful for other Alzheimer's Association Chapters and organizations with related missions are also discussed.

PROBLEMS IN HOSPITAL CARE FOR PERSONS WITH ALZHEIMER'S AND OTHER DEMENTIAS

Over the past ten to fifteen years, many callers to the New York City Chapter's 24-hour telephone Helpline have described distressing situations associated with hospitalization of elderly relatives or friends with Alzheimer's or other dementias. Likewise, in support groups and informational meetings conducted by the Chapter, people with Alzheimer's and other dementias and their families have talked about problems they encountered in emergency room visits, transfers between residential care facilities and hospitals, hospital stays, hospital discharges, and in immediate posthospital periods.

In the spring of 1997, the Chapter newsletter initiated a column entitled, "How It Is: Outrage," by this chapter's coauthor, Jean Marks. The column described the issues that Alzheimer's families were confronting in institutional and hospital care. The following excerpt is from the initial column:

> There is nothing reasonable about Alzheimer's disease. Persons with the disease cannot, can not, adjust to the expectations of institutions. Institutions have to adjust to them.
>
> Alzheimer patients cannot be left alone in emergency rooms. Or examining rooms.
>
> Persons with Alzheimer's disease in the later stages cannot remove the cellophane from dishes on a tray left by their bedside nor feed themselves. They cannot.
>
> Persons with the disease cannot find the dining room in a strange environment; sometimes not in a familiar one.
>
> Persons with Alzheimer's disease cannot tell you where they hurt. If they're frightened.
>
> If they're hungry or need to go to the bathroom.
>
> If they feel lost and confused.
>
> An example: my husband is surprised to find himself in a responsible relationship with a financially successful 83-year old man, not related to us. The man has no real relatives: they were — men, women and children — killed during the Holocaust.
>
> My husband and three other colleagues yearly spend $171,000 trying to obtain the very best care for the old, aphasic man. They make use of one of the "best" nursing homes in the city, a private pay attendant during the day, home care on the weekends, and any and every resource to provide comfort and care for him as they meet other obligations to work and family.
>
> But money cannot buy what the culture does not produce. The old man has been found lying in urine and feces overnight, with re-

cently opened sores on his heels placed on his own body wastes; he has been scheduled by the nursing home for a non-emergency procedure in one of the "best" hospitals, and was left unattended, for 14 hours in the emergency room without food, water, or anyone to tend his needs. A note was pinned on his pajamas that he was unable to talk. No medical records accompanied him. No calls were made to any of his responsible four friends.

If you have had experiences in trying to obtain excellent care for your relative or friend and are livid with indignation at the lack of success, please do submit the incidents to us for this column.

This column, *How It Is*, is not intended to be about bashing any particular institution: home care agencies, nursing homes, and hospitals will not be identified. The column will be about what happens when values are so skewed in a culture that the most common acts of human decency are eclipsed by a more powerful set of assumptions. Those assumptions will, I hope, become visible as we write not of systems, but of individuals — one-by-one — who encounter the systems. They need help, but feel punished for being old and sick (Alzheimer's Association, 1997).

In 2000, the Chapter newsletter presented one family member's story of a difficult emergency room experience. The story, titled "Outrageous," was written by the adult daughter of an elderly woman with dementia who was taken to the emergency room in an ambulance following a fall at home (Alzheimer's Association, 2000). The daughter, a professional geriatric social worker with expertise in Alzheimer's care, reports that she was unable to get accurate information about her mother's condition from emergency room staff; that she was not allowed to see her mother for two hours; that the emergency room staff did not ask her for information about her mother and ignored or rejected her efforts to provide information; that the staff was too quick to use sedatives and physical restraints; and that the staff made medical treatment decisions, claiming that her mother had agreed with the decisions, even though the mother only spoke Spanish and probably could not understand the options presented because of her cognitive impairment. The daughter's feelings of powerlessness, fear, frustration, and anger are clear as she describes her efforts to advocate for her mother in this situation.

Many other families have recounted similar stories and feelings, not only about emergency room care but also about inpatient hospital care. Families have told Chapter staff that they felt ignored and rejected. They have described their concern and anxiety about whether the hospital nurses and aides were aware of their relative's cognitive impairment and sensitive to the special needs that result from it. Many families have said their relative's cognitive and physical status were much worse after discharge than previously and that the person never recovered fully from the hospitalization.

One spouse wrote a column about her husband's hospitalization for tests to determine the cause of blood in his urine. Her husband had been a physician and now could no longer speak or comprehend language. Because he was familiar with the hospital setting, he wanted to leave his room and walk the floors. He was overpowered with a leather restraint and given intravenous Ativan to "calm" him down. When he resisted taking his clothes off, the hospital staff cut them off him, and he was kept restrained with a guard at his door. When the wife arrived to visit, his tray of food was found unopened and untouched; his hands tied to restraints. When he had a bowel accident (because the staff did not respond to a request to untie him and allow him to get to the commode), he became very confused by the four people assigned to clean him up. He hit them; they responded with more restraints and a security guard at his door. He spent days without food or water, until the hospital realized he was dehydrated and they inserted an IV. An enlarged prostate was diagnosed and surgery suggested. Finally, after close to two weeks of being tied down, being poked, given needles, and not given adequate sedation as promised, he was ready to go home. At home he began to re-learn how to eat, but he was becoming very aggressive. The urinary problem started again, and his appetite was poor. It turned out that his aggression was an expression of pain — the only way he could let the world know what he was experiencing, as he had lost all ability to talk. Two months later, he died of undiagnosed cancer of the bladder (Alzheimer's Association, 1998).

As a result of the many disturbing stories about hospital care that have been shared with Chapter staff, staff members often advise families to do anything they can to keep their relative with Alzheimer's or another dementia out of the hospital. Over the years, Chapter staff has also developed relationships with individual physicians and other health care professionals at local hospitals, and they use these contacts to help families whenever they can. Beyond these efforts, however, the Chapter had not initiated specific projects to improve hospital care before it began working with Cabrini Medical Center in 1998. In part, this was because of the many competing demands for Chapter staff time and resources. Weighing more heavily was an additional factor: staff awareness of the likely difficulty of creating meaningful change, especially given the imbalance of power and authority between a large institution with entrenched ideas and practices and a relatively small community agency advocating for changes in care for a small proportion of the hospital's total patient population.

A PLANNING GRANT AND FIRST STEPS TO CHANGE

In 1998, the United Hospital Fund, a foundation in New York City, announced its new "Family Caregiving Grant Initiative" and issued a request for proposals (RFP) for planning grants for local hospitals to clarify their understanding of problems facing family caregivers of hospital patients and to identify potential approaches to address those problems. The next year, the foundation would provide larger grants for hospitals to test the new approaches they had identified in the planning period.

When the New York City Chapter staff read the RFP, they forwarded it the same day to their contacts at local hospitals and offered to work with the hospitals on projects to address problems encountered by family caregivers of people with Alzheimer's and other dementias. Some of the individuals who received the Chapter's message responded that they were not able to undertake a project at that time, but individuals from several hospitals responded positively. The Chapter met with these individuals and eventually submitted joint planning grant proposals with two hospitals, Cabrini Medical Center and the New York University (NYU) Medical Center. Both hospitals received planning grants. This Chapter's work with Cabrini Medical Center is described below. (For a brief description of the NYU project, see Levine, 2003.)

Cabrini, a 500-bed hospital on the lower East side of Manhattan, received the planning grant in May 1998. A project advisory panel was formed with representatives from hospital administration, the hospital's medical and nursing staff, the New York City Chapter, and two family caregivers. Cabrini's planning department director, Allison Braunstein, an organizational psychologist, functioned as the facilitator for the panel. She was instrumental in helping to identify the importance of knowing the root causes of the barriers to providing good care for persons with Alzheimer's disease in the hospitals. Her findings included the following:

1. The system and culture do not support family unit care, empathy, or sympathy.
2. Responsibility for care is diffuse and fragmented.
3. There are too many demands and constraints on time and provision of care.
4. Staff has insufficient education on dementia care and on family unit care.
5. Environmental policies and practices do not support familiarity or caregiver comfort.
6. No mechanism or system exists to collect and disseminate information (especially idiosyncratic information) to all involved.

7. Information written for caregivers does not exist (Cabrini Medical Center, 1998a).

A first step toward addressing these findings was to obtain information to clarify the problems facing family caregivers of hospital patients with Alzheimer's disease and other dementias. For this purpose, three focus groups were conducted with family caregivers. The family caregivers were asked about their experiences with emergency room and hospital care for their relatives and their ideas about what changes were needed to improve hospital care for people with these conditions. Some of the findings from the focus groups are given below:

1. Most caregivers felt that hospital personnel did not communicate with them. The single biggest complaint was that they did not know who to go to with concerns or to ask questions, and that the staff members they did approach were unwilling to respond to them. Most were told to wait for the physician in charge of the patient, even when they asked simple things, and as a result, families spent a lot of "infuriating" time trying to track down the physician, often leaving the facility without resolving their concerns.
2. Few caregivers could recall being asked for information about how to take care of their relatives.
3. Being separated from their relatives in the ER further impeded communication and cut off the caregivers.
4. Interventions by Cabrini religious/spiritual personnel made a significant positive difference through the use of culturally sensitive emotional and spiritual support, but these personnel were often not available when caregivers visited the hospital.
5. No caregivers could recall being asked about or helped with their feelings. (One woman described crying in the ICU and no one paying any attention to her.) Few caregivers were told about support services for themselves, and those that sought out such services did not find them very helpful.
6. Many of the patients' needs were not met well; for example, nobody fed them, nobody addressed the agitation, and nobody could speak to the patient in his or her primary language.
7. The physical facilities were uncomfortable for the caregivers. No caregivers could recall being invited to make it more comfortable, to accommodate themselves overnight, or to bring food or comforting items (Cabrini Medical Center, 1998b).

In addition to the focus groups with family caregivers, Cabrini staff analyzed the hospital's admission procedures to determine sources of stress and uncertainty for patients and families.

Using the findings from the focus groups, the analysis of Cabrini's admissions procedures, and their own perceptions of problems in the way hospitals interact with family caregivers, the project panel attempted to clarify the causes of the problems and identify possible solutions. Lengthy panel meetings were conducted, and the panel members evolved into a cohesive group as they debated these issues.

The skills of the organizational psychologist were paramount to the successful work of the panel. The United Hospital Fund's planning grant provided the "gift of time," but without the leadership of the organizational psychologist, panel members would likely not have been able to do the real work needed for culture change. Under her guidance and with the promise of confidentiality, panel members looked hard at their current relationship with people with Alzheimer's disease and their families. Several hospital staff members had direct experience with Alzheimer's disease as family caregivers; some had experienced hospitalization with their family members. In that atmosphere, the team began to lower organizational turf barriers sufficiently to identify Cabrini's specific problems, to articulate obstacles to better care practices, and to examine Cabrini's history of innovations, including its in-home and inpatient hospice programs and its specialized AIDS unit. The accommodations that hospital staff had made in their effort to create and maintain these innovations were discussed. For the AIDS unit, staff nurses had agreed to make the decision to treat the patients more humanely. Other staff and administration were initially hostile and angry about having to deal with this disease that was not understood. They were afraid of AIDS and felt helpless and impotent in the face of this new plague. These caring nurses agreed to create a "special-care" unit and provide humane, gentle, loving care.

As the summer of 1998 wore on, the Alzheimer's project panel meetings became invigorating. Team members began to reaffirm their individual reasons for wanting to be a health care professional. They began to speak of the potential for alignment of their new goals for patients and families and their own professional and personal values. Eventually, they became committed to a consensual vision of a small, specialized acute care unit in which both the family caregiver and person with Alzheimer's were cared for.

The Alzheimer's Association Chapter representative took a very active role in the panel meetings, contributing to the discussion on several levels. First, she was able to provide expert information and knowledge about Alzheimer's disease and other dementias and the needs of people with these conditions and their family caregivers. She also functioned as a consistent and strong advocate for these people and their families. She also brought family caregivers to the table to share in the discussion and bring their experiences to the panel. Because she was an out-sider to the hospital, she was able to contribute a different perspective than the hospital administrative, medical, and nursing representatives on the panel. When they became entangled in internal organizational is-sues and discouraged about the possibility for change, she could remind them of the project objectives and, equally important, of the hospital's previous success with similar projects that required organizational and culture change and a greater focus on the patient and family as a single unit.

The lengthy panel meetings were valuable. Although all panel members had been aware of some of the problems, their discussions resulted in a deeper and more comprehensive understanding, which was essential for crafting solutions and building the commitment that would be needed to create a new acute care unit. In thinking about the new unit, the panel members recognized that patients with Alzheim-er's and other dementias were being cared for throughout the hospital, but they agreed that it would be too difficult to try to create change on that scale, and that it would be better to focus the change effort on a single unit.

CREATION OF THE "WINDOWS TO THE HEART" UNIT AT CABRINI

Once the decision was made to create a specialized acute care unit for patients with Alzheimer's and other dementias, Cabrini Medical Center applied for the second grant from the United Hospital Fund. The second grant was received in May 1999, and creation of the "Windows to the Heart" unit began. In this second phase, the Chapter continued to pro-vide information and encouragement. When an Alzheimer's care expert was needed to train staff for the new unit, the Chapter identified a psy-chologist with whom they had previously worked. In general, however, the Chapter was less closely involved than it had been during the plan-ning process.

The "Windows to the Heart" unit opened in April 2000. The Chap-ter refers people to the unit and is pleased with the reactions of families who use it. Although other hospitals have specialized geropsychiatry units and acute care units for elderly patients, as of early 2004, the Cabrini unit is still the only specialized acute care unit for patients with Alzheimer's disease and other dementias in the United States. The Chap-ter is proud to have been so extensively involved in the development of this innovative model of hospital care.

NEXT STEPS

Building on the strong working relationship developed over the previous three years, Cabrini Medical Center and the Alzheimer's Association have gone on with two additional projects. In 2002, the Chapter received a grant from the New York City Department for the Aging's "Aging in New York" fund to develop an educational program for use by medical personnel in New York City emergency rooms. The Chapter worked with Jeffrey Nichols, M.D., head of Cabrini's Department of Geriatrics, and delivered five workshops, one in each borough, to emergency room staff. The educational program provided information on (a) recognition of and demonstration of preliminary techniques for diagnosis of cognitive impairment, including possible Alzheimer's disease; (b) recognition of the role the family plays in continuing care post discharge; (c) awareness of in-house social services available to assist in complex cases; and (d) culturally appropriate neighboring services and general referral procedures. The Chapter developed informational posters to be left in the emergency rooms and other materials to remind staff of services in the continuum of care and how to use them. The project was evaluated, and at the time of writing we are awaiting final analysis of the satisfaction and outcome data. (For further information on this project, please contact the first author).

The Chapter also created a volunteer home-visiting program for Cabrini patients with Alzheimer's and other dementias. This Alzheimer's Care Program offers a variety of compassionate services, including creative arts services for persons with Alzheimer's, informational instruction, advocacy, and respite care to give families temporary relief from the burdens of caregiving and allow them to attend to their own needs. The program also offers home visits from a geriatric nurse practitioner who provides health assessments and medical treatment for the person with Alzheimer's disease or other dementias. In April 2003, the Chapter conducted the first of a series of comprehensive trainings about Alzheimer's and dementia for approximately 40 volunteers recruited through Cabrini's Hospice Program. With the nurse practitioner, Chapter staff continues to provide supervision and regular educational updates for those volunteers. As of spring 2004, forty-eight families expressed interest, and thirty families were served by this program in the five boroughs of New York. The program is funded by a Robert Wood Johnson Foundation Faith in Action grant, The United Hospital Fund, and the George Link, Jr. Charitable Trust.

While the New York City Chapter was participating in the planning process for the "Windows to the Heart" unit, Alzheimer's Association

Chapters in other parts of the country became aware of the project and called the Chapter for more information. The Association's national office also created an initiative to improve hospital care for people with dementia. Information, ideas, and professional contacts developed by the New York City Chapter were extremely valuable for the national office initiative. In 1999, when the national office sent out an RFP for a single, $70,000 pilot project on improving hospital care for people with dementia, five large New York City hospitals contacted the Chapter to participate with them in project proposals. The proposed projects included improving nutritional care for hospitalized dementia patients, educating and training hospital staff on Alzheimer's disease, improving transfers from nursing home to acute-care settings for persons with dementia, developing an interactive web-based tutorial for staff, and defining consensual goals for care of hospitalized persons with dementia. Eventually, a small hospital in Oregon was chosen for the grant (see Chapter 8) but the New York City Chapter's work with Cabrini had created widespread interest and enthusiasm among other hospitals in the city. Clearly, the project with Cabrini made a difference beyond that one hospital.

LESSONS FOR OTHER ALZHEIMER'S ASSOCIATION CHAPTERS

The New York City Chapter's work with Cabrini Medical Center provides many lessons that may be useful to other Alzheimer's Association Chapters and organizations with a similar mission and interest in improving the acute care experience for people with Alzheimer's and other dementias. Here are those lessons:

1. People with Alzheimer's and other dementias encounter many difficult and upsetting situations in emergency rooms and hospitals. Although the obstacles to changing this problem are monumental, change is possible.
2. Partnership is essential to create change. Hospitals are complex organizations with many different functions and patient populations to be served. A hospital must understand the problem in its own context and commit to change. On the other hand, a Chapter can help in many ways.
3. In choosing a hospital partner, Chapters should look for hospital administrators and staff who share with the Chapter a common sense of mission and commitment.

4. In choosing a hospital partner, Chapters should consider hospitals that have previously conducted successful projects that required cultural change and a greater emphasis on the patient/family unit and family-centered care, for example, hospitals that changed their maternity units to include fathers, friends, and families in the birth of a baby and hospitals with successful hospice and/or palliative care programs and active bioethics personnel.

5. Although the New York City Chapter worked with a 500-bed hospital (which, in New York City, is a modest size facility), it may be easier to begin with a smaller hospital.

6. Chapters and hospitals should look for outside funding from a foundation or other source. Both Chapters and hospitals are financially strapped at present, and the availability of outside funding will help.

7. It is most important to have a sufficiently lengthy planning period to clarify the aspects of the hospital's existing care practices that are causing problems and identify feasible approaches for change. Such a planning period is time-consuming for everyone involved but essential for a successful project.

8. It is critical to identify and understand the root causes of the problems.

9. In the planning period, the Chapter has many important roles to play, including:

   a. Providing expert information about Alzheimer's disease and other dementias and care for people with these conditions and their families;

   b. Representing and advocating for the people and especially for families, who are generally not a main focus of attention for hospitals;

   c. Offering an outside perspective that can help hospital staff disengage from complex organizational and political pressures (or perhaps see them more clearly) so that they can plan a new program; and

   d. Providing consistent, mission-focused encouragement and support for the planning process and development of the agreed-upon program.

10. Once a strong working relationship has been formed with a hospital, Chapters should use that relationship for additional projects and as a way to reach and influence other hospitals.

11. Chapters should share information and materials from their hospital projects with others in the Chapter network.

BEYOND ACUTE CARE: THE ROLE OF CHAPTERS
AND THE CHAPTER NETWORK

The New York City Chapter of the Alzheimer's Association was established in 1978 by a group of family caregivers. The Chapter was formally incorporated and registered as a nonprofit corporation in New York State in 1985. From the beginning of the Alzheimer's Association, the Chapter network was intended to be an active, responsive presence in communities. An early organizational struggle over which model to use for a new grassroots, single-disease–specific organization resulted in consensus that scarce resources would be put into research and advocacy at a national level and a service component at the local level. The service component, mainly volunteer at first, would concentrate on helping families affected by Alzheimer's disease and related disorders.

The Chapter network became the eyes and ears of the Association and its constituents. Through Helplines, educational forums, and support groups, Chapters were in daily contact with the painful, overwhelming reality caused by the disease and its unrelenting processes. Families talked; Chapters listened and, over time, became increasingly proactive. In some instances, the result has been the creation of a new service, such as the national Safe Return™ program that helps law enforcement personnel return to their caregivers people who wander, become disoriented, and cannot find their way home. In other instances, existing services have been modified sufficiently to make them inclusive of and appropriate for people with Alzheimer's disease and other dementias. For the New York City Chapter, hospice was an early example. The Chapter worked with hospice staff to increase understanding of the dying process for persons with Alzheimer's disease and other dementias. As a result, hospice organizations began to include these people in their services. Working with physicians and researchers at NYU Medical Center, the Chapter helped to create the first prognosticators for end-stage Alzheimer's in the early 1990s; these prognosticators are still in use. Families have been enormously grateful for the physical and psychological care of their family members and themselves. Hospice as it is practiced in New York remains the model service in the hearts and minds of Chapter staff.

The New York City Chapter's work with Cabrini Medical Center illustrates the important role Chapters were intended to play from the beginning. Regardless of the particular service or care setting, this role involves listening to families, understanding their needs, and acting to create change.

In working with institutions such as hospitals, nursing homes, and assisted living facilities, the goal for the New York City Chapter and other Chapters across the country must involve change in the culture of care.

We believe that changing the culture of care for persons with Alzheimer's and other dementias will also benefit others who are vulnerable and cannot advocate for themselves. The shared vision of Chapters across the nation is a collaboration among organizations that represent people with diseases characterized by cognitive impairment, for example, traumatic brain injury, stroke, Parkinson's, and Lupus, to create and sustain culture change in all acute and long-term care institutions and care settings.

CONCLUSION

The Cabrini model works for people with Alzheimer's disease and other dementias. It should be replicated and continuously refined based on new knowledge and experience. Through this model and other approaches, we can support persons with dementia and their families when hospital care is necessary. Hospitalization does not have to be a "nightmare" for all.

When the right combination of forces converges to create change, the project need not be doomed to die of inertia. We remain grateful to the United Hospital Fund for the grant-making model that allowed sufficient time and resources for the project panel to understand the problems in care for persons with Alzheimer's and other dementias, to reach consensus about a solution, and then to implement that solution. Cabrini Medical Center committed itself to this process, participated openly in a comprehensive evaluation of existing care practices, and then established the specialized acute care unit that was envisioned by the panel. The Chapter's role was also essential as catalyst, cheerleader, and spokesperson for the needs of people with dementia and their family caregivers.

While the Alzheimer's Association must certainly continue to support research to find a cure for Alzheimer's disease and other diseases and conditions that cause dementia, the Chapters, the National organization, and our advocacy partners have equally important, ongoing roles to play in listening to families, understanding their needs, and acting to create change. Vulnerable people suffer unnecessarily when we work toward cure and fail to focus sufficiently on the critical issues of changing the culture of care.

REFERENCES

Alzheimer's Association, New York City Chapter. (1997). How it is Outrage. *New York City Alzheimer's Association Chapter Newsletter,* Vol. 14, Spring.

Alzheimer's Association, New York City Chapter. (2000). Outrageous. *New York City Alzheimer's Association Chapter Newsletter,* Vol. 17, Summer.

Alzheimer's Association, New York City Chapter. (1998). How it is: Outrage. *New York City Alzheimer's Association Chapter Newsletter,* Vol. 13, Summer.

Cabrini Medical Center Planning Improvements for Family Caregivers of Minority Dementia Patients Project. (1998a). *Planning summary memorandum: Root causes summary.* New York: Cabrini Medical Center, September 17.

Cabrini Medical Center Planning Improvements for Family Caregivers of Minority Dementia Patients Project. (1998b). *Planning summary memorandum: Findings.* New York: Cabrini Medical Center, September 17.

Levine, C. (2003). *Making room for family caregivers: Seven innovative hospital programs.* New York: United Hospital Fund.

CONCLUSION

Toward a Vision of Dementia-Friendly Hospitals

Nina M. Silverstein and Katie Maslow

Whether the acute care needs of persons with dementia are always best treated in a hospital or could sometimes be more appropriately managed elsewhere in the community is not the question addressed in this book. We have established in Part One that a very large number of persons with dementia, probably at least one-third of all persons with dementia in the United States, are hospitalized each year, and about one-fourth of all elderly hospital patients are persons with dementia. Given current practice patterns and pending a medical breakthrough, that number is likely to increase substantially in coming years as our population ages.

We have illustrated in Part Two that dementia diagnoses frequently are not noted in hospital records, and that dementia is often not recognized or considered at admission, during a person's hospital stay, or in the discharge planning process. Critical information about patients' cognitive status does not get communicated to physicians, nurses, and other front-line hospital staff, nor is this information solicited from family members or other non-hospital care providers. Moreover, the congruence of care and treatment decisions with the preferences and values of the person with dementia is often unknown.

Despite these problems, we conclude that there is reason for optimism. Promising approaches are emerging. Chapters 8, 9, 10, and 11 describe innovative projects that have been implemented in individual hospitals. Chapters 12 and 13 discuss initiatives of the Alzheimer's Association and the John A. Hartford Institute for Geriatric Nursing.

We are also aware of other promising initiatives. A pilot study conducted by the University of Pennsylvania identified many problems faced by people with dementia and their families in the transitional period after discharge from the hospital (Naylor, Stephens, Bowles, & Bixby, 2005). The university has now begun a formal research study to test the effectiveness of an intervention involving advanced practice nurses in addressing these problems. Likewise, Mission Hospitals in Asheville, North Carolina, is conducting a pilot project with the Western Carolina Chapter of the Alzheimer's Association to improve hospital care for people with dementia (Smith-Hunnicutt, 2005).

WHAT WILL IT TAKE FOR HOSPITALS TO DEVELOP AN ORGANIZATIONAL CULTURE AND PRACTICES THAT PROVIDE OPTIMAL CARE FOR PATIENTS WITH DEMENTIA?

Awareness and Support from Senior Hospital Leadership

Improvements in hospital care for people with dementia are unlikely to occur without the understanding and support of senior hospital administrators. While hospital staff members may recognize a general need, the steps between perceived need and action are not often taken until that need is felt in a strong and direct manner by individuals who are in a position to direct change. Given current statistics on the proportion of families that are caring for a relative with dementia, it is likely that many senior hospital administrators will have personally experienced the problems associated with hospitalization for a person with dementia from the vantage point of a family caregiver. Other administrators will have to be convinced of the pressing nature of these problems. Once aware of the problems, these senior leaders will be in a position to serve as catalysts and enablers for system-wide changes in both culture and care practices. Change needs a champion.

Routine Procedures for Recognition of Dementia

Better recognition of dementia is essential for better care. Starting at the time of admission, whether scheduled or unscheduled through the emergency room, hospitals should have in place routine procedures for identifying patients with dementia. These procedures should include asking the person and family (if any) whether the person has a diagnosis of dementia. Since many people with dementia have never been given a formal diagnosis, hospital procedures for recognition of dementia must go beyond this first step. Families should be asked about and staff should be attuned to signs and symptoms of possible dementia that may require further evaluation. Hospital administrators and staff should be aware that recognition of dementia is essential for appropriate care.

Effective Communication about Dementia and Related Care Issues

Once recognized, information about a patient's dementia must be effectively communicated to all hospital personnel who interact with the patient. Communication must go beyond a notation in the person's medical record, and the information must include more that just cognitive status. It should include the person's pre-hospital functional abilities and limitations to guide staff efforts to maintain previous levels of functioning. It should also include, to the extent possible, information about the person's preferences and values with respect to daily care and end-of-life decisions. Family members and other non-hospital care providers are the best source of this information.

Hospital patients are asked many questions. Often they are asked the same questions numerous times as different physicians, nurses, and other personnel gather the information they need to provide care. With recent attention to medical errors, hospital personnel are increasingly pressed to ask some questions over and over. Persons with dementia are very likely to have difficulty responding to questions, and as the number of questions increases, many persons with dementia will become more confused and agitated. Family caregivers, if present, can help with answers to questions. However, these family members will also become upset if repeated questions suggest that hospital personnel are not documenting and sharing the responses. This concern is also relevant for many hospital patients who do not have dementia, but it is especially important for patients with dementia because of their impaired ability to respond accurately and their susceptibility to extreme agitation when confronted with numerous questions they cannot answer.

Once information has been collected and documented in the patient's medical record, the record should be read or the information shared verbally with all hospital personnel who will be responsible for, or involved in, the care of the patient. Red flag information such as "will wander if left unsupervised," "eats finger food only," "does not speak," or "only understands Spanish" should be highlighted and communicated directly to personnel who need the information.

Staff Training in Dementia Care and Strategies for Managing Behavioral Symptoms

There are skills that can be learned and strategies to be shared regarding the care of patients with dementia. Much of the knowledge in this area can be gleaned from best practice experience in caring for persons with dementia in long-term care settings. For example, some long-term care providers have strived for and achieved "restraint-free" care. Likewise, long-term care providers have developed effective ways of managing challenging behaviors.

The *Try This* series developed by the John A. Hartford Institute for Geriatric Nursing and the Alzheimer's Association and described in Chapter 12 is a valuable tool for familiarizing hospital nurses with helpful strategies for caring for patients with dementia. The system-wide approach to training that was implemented at Providence-Milwaukie Hospital and is described in Chapter 8 generated much interest among hospital personnel, increased their awareness of dementia, and provided valuable skills for meeting the acute care needs of cognitively impaired patients. The training for emergency department personnel that was developed by the New York City Chapter of the Alzheimer's Association and medical experts at Cabrini Medical Center bolstered awareness of dementia in the hospitals where it was delivered (Chapters 11 and 13).

Structural Adaptations to Make the Hospital a Dementia-Friendly Environment

Hospital environments can become supportive and often therapeutic through structural changes as well as changes in organizational culture and care practices (Zeisel, Silverstein, Hyde, Levkoff, Lawton, & Holmes, 2003). Administrators and staff at Cabrini Medical Center obtained state-of-the-art recommendations for environmental features that support dementia care when designing the hospital's innovative acute care unit for patients with dementia (Chapter 11).

Discharge Planning That Considers and Accommodates the Patient's Dementia

Discharge planning needs to start early in the hospital stay. Communication with family members and nonhospital care providers who are already involved with the patient's care can provide helpful information for hospital discharge planners. Families and other informal and formal care providers need to be prepared for changes in the patient's functional abilities, whether those changes are short- or long-term. In some instances, hospitalization will trigger a family's first awareness of their relative's cognitive impairments and a first referral for diagnostic evaluation. A hospital stay may also be a time for family members and community care providers to consider, or reconsider, the appropriate care setting for the individual after the acute episode has passed.

A community residence assessment that includes a home visit while the patient is still hospitalized can greatly inform the discharge plan. It is unclear, however, who should conduct the assessment since existing regulations and standards for hospitals and community care providers do not create accountability for successful transitions. Ideally, hospital discharge plans would be based on information about the following questions:

- Can the individual return to his or her prior residence? If the person was previously living with family members or other informal caregivers, are those caregivers able and willing to provide post-hospital and ongoing care? If so, what kinds of help will they need to provide such care?
- If the person was previously living alone, can he or she manage safely in that situation? If yes, is there someone available to assist?
- Was the person driving prior to hospitalization and should his or her driving skills be assessed and monitored? What are the transportation plans for community mobility if driving cessation is necessary?
- If the person was previously living in a nursing home or assisted living facility, is that setting the most appropriate discharge setting?
- Do modifications need to be made to the home or assisted living residence?
- Should a short-term rehabilitation center be considered?
- Does the individual require skilled nursing care and is new, nursing home placement warranted?

- If medications are prescribed, what are the pláns for assistance with medication management?

Effective Ways of Connecting Patients and Their Families to Supportive Community Services

Supportive services are available in many communities, but the patient and his or her family may not be aware of these services or understand how the services relate to their individual needs. Since hospital discharge planners have limited time to keep up-to-date information about community services for persons with dementia, the one-stop-shopping contact that discharge planners should identify is the Alzheimer's Association.

The Alzheimer's Association is a voluntary health organization dedicated to finding preventions, treatments and eventually, a cure for Alzheimer dementia. It has a nationwide network of chapters that offer a broad range of programs and services for people with the disease, families,and care partners (Alzheimer's Association, 2004a) Local chapters of the Alzheimer's Association may be found by visiting: www.alz. org.

Chapter 2 notes that the Safe Return™ program, a wanderers' alert program sponsored by the Justice Department in association with the Alzheimer's Association, was not well known by a sample of patient care directors in Massachusetts. Awareness of this program would be helpful to hospital staff who could benefit by learning prevention strategies for minimizing harmful consequences of unsafe wandering and protocols to follow during an elopement episode. Awareness of the program would also help family caregivers who could be given information about Safe Return™ at the time of hospital discharge. Information about support groups for the individuals, their caregivers, their children, and their grandchildren could also be shared at the time of discharge. Providence-Milwaukie Hospital placed brochures from the Alzheimer's Association chapter in kiosks throughout the hospital and had to replenish them frequently (Chapter 8).

Another more general one-stop-shopping for community-based care is through the *Eldercare Locator,* a national toll-free referral number funded by the U.S. Administration on Aging (AoA) to help older people and their families find community services for seniors anywhere in the country. *Eldercare Locator* is administered by the National Association of Area Agencies on Aging in cooperation with the National Association of State Units on Aging and is intended to connect callers to the best state and community sources of information and assistance to address the issues, needs, or concerns of older persons and their caregivers. The Web site for *Eldercare Locator* is: http://www.n4a.org/locator.cfm.

Geriatric care managers (Chapter 5) are another critical partner in community care, particularly when family caregivers are not available. These are social workers, nurses, or case managers who may be associated with public agencies or private practices and who coordinate care for the elder in the community. Geriatric care managers are also helpful in mediating family conferences either in-person or among long-distance caregivers.

Adult day services can help to keep persons with dementia safe in the community. Adult day centers provide supervised activities in a safe environment and often offer transportation to and from the person's residence while the primary caregiver is at work. Discharge planners should become familiar with local adult day health centers.

Assisted living residences have become home to many persons with dementia. It is estimated that approximately half of residents aged 65+ in assisted living, including both dementia-specific and general assisted living residences, have dementia (Alzheimer's Association, 2004b). Discharge planners, if not already familiar, should become familiar with the assisted living residences in their communities that serve the special needs of persons with dementia. Since the level of care required by some persons with dementia is beyond the services available through assisted living, discharge planners should also be aware of local nursing homes that provide appropriate care for residents with dementia.

FINAL THOUGHTS

The message in the multiple perspectives shared in this book is that persons with dementia find themselves hospitalized for their acute care needs and often leave the hospital in worse shape than when they entered, having lost preadmission functional abilities. Strategies for acknowledging dementia and managing challenging behaviors were presented in almost every chapter. Implementation of any of these strategies would be a positive step toward improving hospital care for the patient with dementia.

REFERENCES

Alzheimer's Association. (2004a). Retrieved December 22, 2004, from http:// www.alz.org/AboutUs/overview.asp

Alzheimer's Association. (2004b). People with Alzheimer's disease and dementia in assisted living. Advocacy and Public Policy Division. Retrieved December 23, 2004, from http://www.alz.org/Advocacy/downloads/prevalence_ Alz_assist.pdf

Naylor, M. D., Stephens, C., Bowles, K. H., & Bixby, M. B. (2005). Cognitively impaired older adults: From hospital to home: An exploratory study of these patients and their caregivers. *American Journal of Nursing 105*(2): 52–61.

Smith-Hunnicutt, N. Dementia-responsive acute care at Mission Hospitals in Asheville, North Carolina. (2005). *North Carolina Medical Journal, 66*(1): 72–74.

Zeisel, J., Silverstein, N.M., Hyde, J., Levkoff, S., Lawton, M.P., & Holmes, W. (2003). Environmental correlates to behavioral outcomes in Alzheimer's special care units. *The Gerontologist, 43*, 697–711.

Index

Page numbers followed by f or t indicate figures or tables.

A Guide for
Nursing Home Social Workers

Elise M. Beaulieu, MSW, ACSW, LICSW

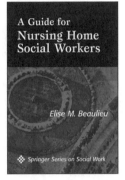

"In this excellent volume on social work practice in nursing homes, the author presents an in-depth discussion of all aspects of nursing home practice. ...The book is essential reading for beginning and experienced social workers alike. It is also an outstanding text for courses that include content on practice in long term care."

—Patricia Brownell, PhD, CSW
Fordham University Graduate School of Social Service

This book clearly distinguishes the function of beginning nursing home social workers and provides information and resources essential for them. Topics include the following: the assessment, intake, and discharge processes; interventions; resource allocation; medication; diagnosis and treatment of depression; dementias; and legal issues, ethics, and confidentiality agreements. Making the volume still more practical are a glossary of commonly used terms and abbreviations, as well as a section of standardized forms and charts.

Contents:

- Basic Orientation
- Social Work in Nursing Facilities
- The Nursing Facility
- Surveys
- Diagnoses and Treatment
- Legal Representatives for Residents
- Ethics
- Community Liaisons
- Problems and Solutions
- Sample Forms

Social Work Series
2002   304pp   0-8261-1533-0   softcover

11 West 42nd Street, New York, NY 10036-8002 • Fax: 212-941-7842
Order Toll-Free: 877-687-7476 • Order On-line: www.springerpub.com

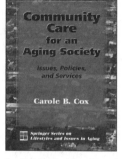

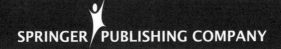

SPRINGER PUBLISHING COMPANY

End-of-Life Stories
Crossing Disciplinary Boundaries
Donald E. Gelfand, PhD, Richard Raspa, PhD
Sherylyn H. Briller, PhD
Stephanie Myers Schim, PhD, RN, APRN, CNAA, BC, Editors

This book provides a variety of narratives about end-of-life experiences contributed by members of the Wayne State University End-of-Life Interdisciplinary Project. Each of the narratives is then analyzed from three different disciplinary perspectives. These analyses broaden how specific end-of-life narratives can be viewed from different dimensions and help students, researchers, and practitioners see the important and varied meanings that end-of-life experiences have at the level of the individual, the family, and the community. In addition, the narratives include end-of-life experiences of individuals from a variety of ethnic and racial backgrounds.

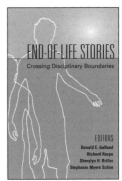

Partial Contents:

2005   218pp   0-8261-2675-8   hardcover

11 West 42nd Street, New York, NY 10036-8002 • Fax: 212-941-7842
Order Toll-Free: 877-687-7476 • Order On-line: www.springerpub.com